Instructor's Manual to Accompany

NUTRITION
Essentials and Diet Therapy

Seventh Edition

Nancy J. Peckenpaugh, MSEd, RD, CDE

Dietitian in Private Practice
Lifetime Nutrition Services
Ithaca, New York

Charlotte M. Poleman, BS, RD

Community Dietitian
Broome Developmental Services
Ithaca, New York

W.B. SAUNDERS COMPANY

A Division of Harcourt Brace & Company
Philadelphia London Toronto
Montreal Sydney Tokyo

W.B. Saunders Company
A Division of
Harcourt Brace & Company

The Curtis Center
Independence Square West
Philadelphia, PA 19106

Instructor's Manual to Accompany
Nutrition: Essentials and Diet Therapy
Seventh Edition

ISBN   0-7216-5131-3

Printed in the United States of America

Last digit is the print number: 9 8 7 6 5 4 3 2 1

TABLE OF CONTENTS

We are happy to provide this *Instructor's Manual* to assist the instructors using Peckenpaugh and Poleman: *Nutrition: Essentials and Diet Therapy, Seventh Edition*, in the classroom or clinical setting. This resource includes a wealth of teaching tools both for the new instructor and for the experienced instructor looking for new approaches to teaching:

- Sample test questions (mostly multiple-choice format)
- Suggestions for using the on-going case study in the text, "A Family's Perspectives on Nutrition"
- Answers to study questions and activities found in the textbook
- Suggested reading and audiovisual aids specific to the individual chapter; ordering information is included in these listings
- Overhead transparency masters
- Contact information for other sources of nutrition-related information

The authors recommend that the student and instructor keep abreast of current nutrition literature. There are continual advances in the science and art of nutrition with which no textbook can keep up. Reading nutrition journals such as *The Journal of the American Dietetic Association, Nutrition Today, The American Journal of Clinical Nutrition*, and the *Journal of Nutrition Education* will assist the instructor and student in keeping informed of new developments in the field of nutrition.

Nutrition: Essentials and Diet Therapy, Seventh Edition is based on some general objectives that we feel are appropriate for the students who will use the text as a learning and reference tool. These objectives can be grouped in terms of attitude, knowledge, and skills.

Attitude. Insofar as nutrition is a holistic clinical science that comprehends many aspects of individual and societal life, the *attitude* exhibited by the health care worker is crucial and is most effective when it reflects:

- An appreciation of the role of nutrition for optimal health, efficiency, longevity, and enjoyment of life for everyone, including oneself and one's family.
- An understanding of the importance of the right kinds and amounts of foods to be eaten daily for good nutrition.
- A recognition of the role of nutrition in the total care of the patient—that is, to maintain good nutrition when necessary, or to use a single nutrition therapeutic measure or as one of several modalities.
- An appreciation of the social, ethnic, religious, economic, and psychological factors, as well as the physiological factors, in feeding both well and ill persons.
- An understanding of the patient's established patterns of eating.
- An appreciation of the importance of having the right attitude toward food and nutritional habits for success in feeding patients and in obtaining their willingness to accept dietary modifications.
- An appreciation of the importance of the normal basic diet as a foundation for any therapeutic modification.
- An appreciation of the health care professional's role and responsibility in educating patients and their families, as well as community members, in good nutritional habits.

Knowledge. Even at its simplest, nutrition is a complex science, requiring constant review and updating of one's own information base, particularly regarding:

- The characteristics of adequate and inadequate nutritional status.
- The nutrients necessary for good nutrition and their function in the body.
- The nutritional values of foods in the various food groups.
- The nutritional needs of individuals in different age groups and under varying conditions.
- The daily food guides for good nutrition.

- The ways in which the normal diet is modified for therapeutic purposes (now referred to as "medical nutrition therapy").
- The principles of meal planning for nutritional adequacy and palatability.
- Common food fads and fallacies.
- The agencies concerned with problems of nutrition and health.
- Diseases that require dietary modification and what is involved in medical nutrition therapy.
- The basic relationships between foods and medications.

Skills. Because nutrition is a clinical science, the continuing development of one's clinical techniques is crucial and involves:

- The ability to recognize outward signs of good and poor nutrition.
- The ability to apply basic principles of nutrition to the wise selection of daily foods for oneself and one's family.
- The ability to serve food attractively and in the correct amounts.

- The ability to make simple modifications in the normal diet to conform to the physician's therapeutic dietary order or to adapt a family meal for the family member requiring medical nutrition therapy.
- The ability to answer patients' questions regarding food and nutrition and help them understand the reasons for their nutritional therapy and the need for their cooperation.
- The ability to report to the physician and dietitian about a patient's dietary problems or needs.
- The ability to give a patient assistance at mealtimes.
- The ability to advise on nutritional care at home.
- The ability to evaluate the adequacy of meals consumed at home or in an institutional setting.

The authors invite suggestions and comments regarding both the text and *Instructor's Manual.* Please write to us in care of the W. B. Saunders Company, Nursing Department.

INTRODUCTION TO NUTRITION AND A MULTICULTURAL CASE STUDY MINISERIES

SAMPLE TEST QUESTIONS

Match the letter of the term in Column B with the appropriate term in Column A

A

_____ 1. Nutritional status (f)

_____ 2. Nutritional care (d)

_____ 3. Dietitian (e)

_____ 4. Health (b)

_____ 5. Public health (a)

_____ 6. Holistic health (c)

B

a. Field of medicine

b. More than the absence of disease

c. Preventive medicine that takes into account the whole individual

d. Application of nutrition knowledge

e. Nutritionist

f. Condition of the body as it relates to the consumption and use of food

---

7. Carbohydrate is:
   a. a quick and easy energy source *
   b. a stored, long-lasting energy source
   c. good for building muscles
   d. found in butter and margarine

8. The following phrase describes the interplay of external and internal forces on health:
   a. nutritional status
   b. biopsychosocial conerns *
   c. health care team
   d. none of the above

9. Although health may be restored without medicine, it cannot be maintained without proper:
   a. nutrition *
   b. transportation
   c. lab tests
   d. none of the above

10. Which of the following is not a part of the health care team:
    a. the patient
    b. the doctor
    c. the dietitian
    d. none of the above *

11. To be effective in helping an individual make dietary changes the following is important:
    a. displaying warmth and understanding
    b. establishing a rapport with the person
    c. focusing on positive messages
    d. all of the above *

12. The following health concerns tend to have a genetic link:
    a. obesity and hypertension
    b. atherosclerosis and hyperlipidemia
    c. various forms of cancer
    d. all of the above *

13. A change to a Westernized diet and lifestyle increases the risk of obesity and diabetes among several ethnic groups:
    a. true *
    b. false

14. Diabetes, lactose intolerance, and food allergies do not tend to run in families:
    a. true
    b. false *

15. There are more than 50 nutrients needed by the body:
    a. true *
    b. false

INSTRUCTIONAL POINTS ON "A FAMILY'S PERSPECTIVE ON NUTRITION"

Not applicable

ANSWERS TO TEXTBOOK STUDY QUESTIONS AND ACTIVITIES

1. Those who have a knowledge of the science of nutrition are able to interpret and determine a person's nutritional needs in both health and disease and can help the public become aware of myths and misconceptions about nutrition that are common in our society today.

2. Many factors affect a person's state of health, including:
   - Proper functioning of all body parts
   - Good posture
   - Good health and hygiene habits
   - Good mental attitude
   - Correction of remediable defects

3. The three functions of food are to:
   - Provide energy
   - Build and maintain body cells
   - Regulate body processes

4. Four skills are needed to apply knowledge about nutrition:
   - Ability to recognize outward signs of good and poor nutrition
   - Ability to apply basic principles of nutrition to the wise selection of foods for oneself and one's family
   - Ability to plan adequate and palatable meals for oneself and one's family
   - Ability to assist in the planning and implementation of methods for the achievement of nutritional goals

5. Some ethnic foods the class may want to research for nutritional content:
   - Grits (Southern U.S.)—usually served as hot cereal (corn based)
   - Hopping John (Southern U.S)—a dish with black-eyed peas and rice
   - Bangers and Mash (British)—mashed potatoes, sausage link, and gravy
   - Moo Goo Gai Pan (Chinese)—a chicken dish
   - Spanokopita (Greek)—phyllo dough filled with spinach and cheese
   - Pasta Fazula (Italian)—a pasta and bean soup
   - Frijoles (Mexico)—staple dish of beans
   - Cassava Pie (Bermuda)—a chicken-filled pie made with cassava flour

6. Have students list family health problems and list of known heritage such as British, French, German, Italian, Greek, African, Indian, Mexican, Chinese, and so on. Are there any patterns noted by the class such as lactose-intolerance, diabetes, obesity, and the like. (This exercise should be optional as students may not want to discuss heritage or family health issues with classmates.)

AUDIOVISUAL AIDS AND SUGGESTED READING

ETHNIC COOKING. Produced by Holloway Productions. Five separate videotapes and teacher's guides each for $49.00 ($169.00 for the complete set of five VHS videotapes). Tapes include presentations of geographic location, cultural heritage, climatic conditions, and typical eating habits in the respective countries. Step-by-step cooking techniques with reproducible recipes are provided in the instructor's guide. The programs are: Chinese Cuisine, Provincial French Cuisine, Scandanavian Cuisine, Italian Cuisine, and Mexican Cuisine. Order from: NASCO, 901 Janesville Ave., Fort Atkinson, Wisconsin 53538-0901 or call 1-800-558-9595 or fax 414-563-8296.

ETHNIC CUISINE. Produced by Holloway Productions. Three separate 20-minute videotapes with written recipes and teacher's guides. Similar in format to the above Ethnic Cooking series. Cuisines covered include African-American Cuisine, Greek Cuisine, and German Cuisine. Price: $69.00 each or $154.00 for the complete set on one videotape. Order from NASCO (see ordering information above).

FOOD REPLICAS, REALISTIC ETHNIC FOODS. Ethnic food models include Mexican-American foods, American Foods of the South, and Italian foods. Foods sold separately from the NASCO catalog. To order the catalog use the above address.

BETTER HOMES AND GARDEN COOKING ITALIAN. Illustrated, 128 pages. Price: $12.95. Order from NASCO using the above address.

BETTER HOMES AND GARDENS, COOKING CHINESE and ORIENTAL COOKBOOK. Both cookbooks illustrated. Price: $9.95 each. Order from NASCO using the above address.

NUTRITION IN A FAMILY MEAL ENVIRONMENT

CHAPTER 1

SAMPLE TEST QUESTIONS

1. The USDA Food Guide Pyramid shows:
   a. minimum levels for preventing chronic diseases
   b. how the Dietary Guidelines are incorporated into five food groups *
   c. animal food sources should be a large part of the total diet
   d. plant foods are a small part of the total diet

2. An example of external barriers to adequate nutrient intakes are:
   a. lack of food storage facilities
   b. inadequate money to purchase food
   c. lack of exposure to a variety of foods
   d. all of the above *

3. Americans, in general, are eating:
   a. more sugar than 100 years ago *
   b. more meat since the 1970s
   c. plenty of fruits and vegetables as recommended by health experts
   d. higher fat diets

4. Ethnic eating habits indicate:
   a. Chinese have lower blood cholesterol levels than Americans due to eating less cholesterol and saturated fat *
   b. The French eat more shortening, oil, eggs, and sugar than Americans
   c. Greeks and Southern Italians have high rates of heart disease
   d. Japanese have a high cancer risk

5. In the lacto-ovo vegetarian diet:
   a. dairy products and eggs are excluded
   b. dairy foods and eggs supplement plant foods *
   c. fish and chicken are never included
   d. there are inadequate amounts of nutrients and this diet should never be followed

6. In planning a vegetarian diet the following principles should be used:
   a. emphasis on a wide variety of plant foods
   b. increase intake of legumes
   c. intake of nutrient-dense foods
   d. all of thc above *

7. Fast foods are:
   a. junk foods
   b. not good to eat in a balanced meal plan
   c. unhealthy
   d. able to meet the criteria of the USDA Type A school lunch program *

Match the letter of the term in Column B with the appropriate term in Column A

A	**B**
____ 8. milkshakes, milk (b)	a. complex carbohydrates
____ 9. orange juice, coleslaw (f)	b. high in calcium and phosphorus
____ 10. enriched rolls, french fries (a)	c. empty kcalories
____ 11. soft drinks (c)	d. protein rich
____ 12. fish, chicken, beef, cheese (d)	e. rich source of fat
____ 13. mayonnaise, french fries (e)	f. vitamin C

Match the letter in Column B with the appropriate term in Column A

A	**B**
____ 14. beta carotene (c)	a. several forms found in all plant foods
____ 15. chronic disease (d)	b. dried beans and peas
____ 16. grazing (f)	c. turns to vitamin A in the body
____ 17. fiber (a)	d. any disease of long standing
____ 18. legumes (b)	e. caused by lack of iodine
____ 19. goiter (e)	f. frequent all-day eating

---

20. Empty kcalories
    a. provide simple carbohydrate and fat *
    b. are inappropriate for maintenance of ideal weight
    c. contribute protein, vitamins, and minerals
    d. are harmful even on an occasional basis

INSTRUCTIONAL POINTS ON "A FAMILY'S PERSPECTIVE ON NUTRITION"

- Have students discuss their own family environments. Can anyone relate to the Bernardo family as described? Are there any students with Italian heritage that can expand on food and nutrition issues of American-Italian families? Are there any students with other ethnic backgrounds that can tell a similar or unique story?
- Have students reflect on what culture means. Can food habits be equated to other forms of cultures; i.e., have students describe how the food choices of a teenaged population might differ from an elderly population. How might this impact on nutrition advice? Brainstorm other subcultures such as religious groups or sports groups and how food choices might be affected.
- Have students reflect on the amount of meat consumed in the United States versus other countries of the world. Can the students describe how U.S. food culture has promoted obesity, heart disease, and hypertension?
- Have students describe their usual meal settings at home and how this experience may impact on their attitudes toward good nutritional habits. Did they have sit-down meals? Were meal times pleasant? Was food used as a reward; such as dessert? Were there adequate amounts of healthy food choices in their homes?
- Have students do an informal 5-minute observation of the types of people that go to a fast food restaurant i.e., have them count the number of children with parents, older children without parents at the restaurant, the number of women versus men, the number of people who appear to be past the retirement age, and so on.

ANSWERS TO TEXTBOOK STUDY QUESTIONS AND ACTIVITIES

1. Good meal planning is a science in that it can be quantified in tools such as the RDAs, the basic five food groups of the Food Guide Pyramid, and exchange lists so that research on nutritional impact is possible. As an art, meal planning includes understanding the subtle influences of meal environment (such as attitudes, cultural influences, religious influences, and other environmental factors) on nutritional intake and knowing strategies to facilitate positive meal environments and nutritional intake.

2. Potential nutritional problems of the Bernardo family include:
   - Reliance on convenience foods due to a hectic lifestyle
   - High intake of sodium and fat from snack food choices
   - Inadequate nutritional intake due to lower income
   - Overweight of the teenaged daughter, Anna
   - Underweight of the teenaged son, Joey

   To assist the Bernardo family in meeting their health and nutrition needs:
   - Evaluate the nutritional intake of carbohydrate, protein, fat, vitamins, and minerals
   - Determine individual nutrition concerns and eating practices
   - Suggest eating at least the minimum number of food servings of the Food Guide Pyramid with emphasis on foods low in saturated fat, sugar, and sodium

   Potential questions to assess their nutritional intake and status:
   - What foods are commonly eaten for meal times and snacks?
   - What are the height and weight of family members? Any significant increases or decreases in weight?

   If you assess that high fat/high sodium convenience foods are chosen for meals and snacks interventions might include reading labels (see Chapter 6) and substituting low fat/low sodium snacks such as low-salt pretzels, bagels, fruit, and so on.

3. Vitamin A snacks —carrot sticks, watermelon wedge, canteloupe (melon balls), dried apricots, broccoli flowerets, pumpkin pie

   Vitamin C snacks—citrus juice, orange wedges, strawberries, green pepper slices, cauliflowerets, tomato juice

   Calcium —milk, yogurt, pudding, cheese, soymilk, almonds, sardines

Iron—iron-fortified cereals, nuts and raisins, whole-grain crackers or toast, black-strap molasses (mixed in a glass of milk or spread on peanut butter toast or added to baked goods in place of some sugar)

4. Small hamburger   Pizza slice with
    Low-fat milk   lean meat
    Tossed salad with   Fruit salad
       oil and vinegar   Carrot sticks
    Orange juice

5. Effective strategies to overcome food dislikes or avoidances include:
    • Repeated tasting as tastes are learned
    • Using food in different ways such as carrots in carrot bread or carrot and raisin salad, stew with carrots, shredded carrots or carrot curls, soup with carrots

6. If the Bernardo children became vegetarians it would be important to promote whole grains and legumes. If they would drink milk and eat eggs adequate amounts of protein would easily be obtained.

7. Magazine food ads—look for sex appeal and how foods are promoted (nutritional, appearance, taste, as a reward, i.e., "go ahead, you deserve it" or other reasons). Observe other features of the people in the ad such as gender, age, and style of clothes (suit or blue jeans and so on)

8.

Diet	Characteristics	Good Features	Desirable Changes
Jewish	Kosher meats and other foods (marked with a K or a U in a circle on many common foods); meat not eaten with dairy	Includes all food groups (milk and cheese can be in the meat group)	Use low-fat milk products; include high iron foods if meat is restricted along with vitamin C foods for iron absorption
Chinese	Little meat or milk with emphasis on fish, eggs, rice, and vegetables	High in complex carbohydrate, meets five food groups if tofu is eaten (a milk substitute), low in fat and high in vitamins A and C	Use lactose-reduced milk if tolerated to increase calcium intake, use low-sodium soy sauce
Southern U. S.	Includes many meats such as chicken, ham, pork, variety meats (fish in coastal areas; red meat inland); corn bread, grits, greens, black-eyed peas, sweet potatoes, pecans	Can be high in fiber and vitamins A and C; meets basic five food groups; salsa (a low fat topping), mayonnaise (low in saturated fat)	Use less saturated fats such as bacon fat and butter; use less total fat; emphasize beans and lean meat
Great Britain	Meats include lamb, kidneys, fish such as finian haddie, salt cod, and salmon; potatoes and turnip; afternoon tea with tarts or other sweet biscuits, cake or Scottish Bread; Marmite (a salty beef based spread used on toast)	Meets basic food groups, generally low in meat portions (a "British" sandwich contains only about 1 ounce of meat)	Use low-fat milk, less butter; emphasize fish and vegetables with less total fat intake; use lower fat and lower sugar biscuits such as "Digestive Biscuits" or small portions of high-fat baked goods; use thin spread of Marmite

AUDIOVISUAL AIDS AND SUGGESTED READING

SNACK ATTACKS ARE OKAY. A client education pamphlet discusses who needs to snack, myths and facts concerning snacking, and snacks in a variety of everyday situations. A package of 25—price: $4.89 ($4.00 for ADA members). Available from The American Dietetic Association, 216 W. Jackson Blvd., Chicago, IL 60606-6995 or call 312/899-0040.

EATING WELL—THE VEGETARIAN WAY. A client education pamphlet describes various forms of vegetarianism and provides guidelines for healthful vegetarian meals for adults and children. A package of 25—price: $4.89 ($4.00 for ADA members). Available from The American Dietetic Association (see above ordering information).

THE NUTRITION CARE PROCESS AS USED BY HEALTH CARE PROFESSIONALS

CHAPTER 2

SAMPLE TEST QUESTIONS

1. The nutrition care process:
   a. includes assessment, planning, intervention, education, and diagnosis
   b. uses non-verbal communication only
   c. is the same as the nursing process with the omission of diagnosis *
   d. steps do not have to be followed in order

2. Nutritional assessments include:
   a. the client's initial medical and nutritional status
   b. psychological issues
   c. knowledge of previous health concerns
   d. all of the above *

3. The Health Belief Model:
   a. is based on the theory that a patient will make health decisions in line with personal health values and "costs" versus benefits of changes to be made *
   b. is based on the fact that a person's motivation to make lifestyle changes should not be determined prior to the intervention phase
   c. cannot help the person evaluate his or her health beliefs
   d. tries to show that changing lifestyle will provide psychological benefits

---

Match the letter of the term in Column B with the appropriate term in Column A

A

_____ 4. active listening (f)

_____ 5. change agent (e)

_____ 6. cognitive (d)

_____ 7. Health Belief Model (a)

_____ 8. affective (c)

_____ 9. albumin (b)

B

a. perceived benefits versus cost

b. to determine protein status

c. attitudes

d. knowledge

e. one who helps patients make changes in lifestyle

f. nonjudgmental type of questioning

10. Planning strategies:
    a. do not include input by the patient
    b. include "I" statements to make recommendations sound less threatening *
    c. do not depend on goals and rationale for change
    d. avoid a time frame for achieving goals

11. Mr. Bernardo:
    a. did not know his wife was pregnant when he went to see his doctor about his lab results
    b. had a low hemoglobin level
    c. had a minimum wage job *
    d. needed surgery

12. The evaluation of outcomes:
    a. may be based on quizzes as appropriate
    b. may involve monitoring lab values
    c. may be done through formal or informal conversation
    d. all of the above *

13. Tony Bernardo, the Italian-American person described in the opening chapter case study, did not have to worry about heart disease since there is little heart disease in Italy:
    a. true
    b. false *

14. Health care professionals should be aware of local support services and health professionals specializing in diabetes for referral purposes:
    a. true *
    b. false

15. Which of the following is an example of a good active-listening question:
    a. "Here is a diet sheet provided by a pharmaceutical company."
    b. "You are wrong, let me tell you what is right."
    c. "How do you feel about eating less fat and sugar?" *
    d. "Who do you know that can help you?"

INSTRUCTIONAL POINTS ON "A FAMILY'S PERSPECTIVE ON NUTRITION"

- Have students discuss how recent and past experiences might impact on a person's receptivity to a diagnosis such as diabetes. For example, Mr. Bernardo's recent stressful life events (loss of job, wife pregnant, running late to his doctor's appointment). How might Mr. Bernardo cope with the diagnosis if he has had a family history of diabetes with complications versus not knowing anything about the impact of the disease?

- Have the students imagine they were in Donna's place (Dr. Shaw's new nurse). Would they be nervous about the encounter? How might their feelings and actions affect how Mr. Bernardo feels?

- Discuss how Dr. Shaw's taking a few deep breaths to relax himself before he faced Mr. Bernardo could positively affect the outcome of this patient encounter. What might happen in this patient session if he focused on all the negative aspects of diabetes management, i.e., all the adverse complications of diabetes if he won't make appropriate lifestyle changes.

ANSWERS TO TEXTBOOK STUDY QUESTIONS AND ACTIVITIES

1. Donna could use the following assessment questions with Mr. Bernardo:
   - "How are you today?"
   - "Do you have any further questions now that Dr. Shaw has explained your diagnosis?"
   - "Is there anything more we can do for you today?"

2. Dr. Shaw probably thought of referral sources for diabetes management for Mr. Bernardo because:
   - He recognizes that there will be many questions and emotions that Mr. Bernardo will need to process.
   - A registered dietitian, especially one who is a certified diabetes educator, can help Mr. Bernardo develop a meal plan and eating strategies that will allow for permanent dietary changes to control blood sugar and lipid levels.
   - A social worker can help Mr. Bernardo with community assistance programs due to a low-paying job and his high health expenses related to his wife's pregnancy and his diabetes management. The social worker can also help him sort through his many emotions that would be expected upon learning of his chronic disease.

- A smoking cessation support group can help smokers to stop and are often run free or at a nominal fee.

3. Questions that may be used by Dr. Shaw to assess Tony's health belief system regarding diabetes management are:
   - "Can you tell me what you know about diabetes?"
   - "How do you feel about eating less sugar and fat and increasing exercise?"
   - "How do you feel about eating more soluble fiber sources such as beans?"
   - "Is aiming for at least a 10 to 15 pound weight loss realistic for you?"
   - "Do you think you're likely to read labels for sodium content of foods?"
   - "How would you feel if I referred you to see a dietitian to arrange a meal plan?"
   - "A social worker can help you sort out your feelings and give you guidance on community resources to manage diabetes and finances; how would you feel about seeing one?"
   - "Can I talk you into a smoking-cessation support group?"

4. No, Dr. Shaw should not start his session with Mr. Bernardo by discussing all of the adverse health outcomes related to poor diabetes management. This sets too negative a tone when he first has to deal with the shock of having a chronic illness. Doing so may promote a denial reaction as it can be easier to deal with this recognition by blocking it out of the mind. Understanding the basic mechanics of the disease and its treatment with emphasis on making positive small steps is the best approach. Long-term complications should only be alluded to at the first visit.

5. No, Dr Shaw's nurse, Donna, was correct not to discuss Mr. Bernardo's diagnosis on the telephone. This is the role of the doctor.

6. Encourage the students to use active-listening techniques as discussed in the text when they are doing the role-play (as used by the nurse or other health professional). Have other class members list examples of open-ended and close-ended questions as used by the "health care professional." Have students discuss their reactions after the role-play, both the "nurse" and the "patient." A role-play volunteer may elect to play Mr. Bernardo, make up their own character, or act as herself or himself.

AUDIOVISUAL AIDS AND SUGGESTED READING

WORKSITE NUTRITION: A GUIDE TO PLANNING, IMPLEMENTATION, AND EVALUATION, 2nd ed. This publication outlines general planning, implementation, and evaluation strategies to encourage healthful eating in both small and large organizations. Price: $12.00 ($10.00 for ADA members). Available from The American Dietetic Association, 216 W. Jackson Blvd., Chicago, IL 60606-6995 or call 312/899-0040.

DEVELOPING HEALTH EDUCATION MATERIALS FOR SPECIAL AUDIENCES: LOW-LITERATE ADULTS, 1992. By J.E. Shield and M.C. Mullen. An audiotape program with printed study guide that focuses on the three-phase process of planning, developing, and evaluating health education materials for low-literate adults. Audiotape and study guide price: $39.95 ($34.00 ADA members). Available from The American Dietetic Association (see above ordering information).

LEARNING THROUGH LAUGHTER, 1990. By R. Flipse. Shows how humor can help get nutrition messages across on subjects such as food labels, diet fads, and diet and heart disease. Featured are suggestions for use and information on reproducing copyrighted material. Price: $12.65 ($11.00 ADA members). Order from ADA (see above).

CARBOHYDRATE, PROTEIN, AND FAT: THE ENERGY MACRONUTRIENTS OF BALANCED MEALS

CHAPTER 3

SAMPLE TEST QUESTIONS

1. The macronutrients of food:
   a. are not essential for life
   b. include carbohydrate, protein, and fat *
   c. provide 9 kcalories per gram
   d. provide 4 kcalories per gram

2. The base of the diet should:
   a. emphasize protein foods
   b. emphasize plant foods *
   c. emphasize simple carbohydrates
   d. provide 30% of the total kcalories in the diet

3. Carbohydrates:
   a. are formed by all green plants through photosynthesis *
   b. are composed of only carbon and hydrogen
   c. cause dental caries in the presence of a clean mouth
   d. all of the above

4. The term biological value describes:
   a. how much protein the body needs daily
   b. the only way vegetarians can receive adequate protein
   c. how much of the essential amino acids that a food contains *
   d. none of the above

5. Amino acids:
   a. can all be synthesized by the human body
   b. can be found in varying amounts and combinations in the foods we eat *
   c. are not necessary for the formation of enzymes
   d. do not contain carbon

6. Protein:
   a. is essential for life *
   b. requirement is always increased during long convalescence
   c. allowance is less per kg body weight during childhood
   d. in excess leads to an increased need for vitamins and minerals

7. Fats:
   a. contain 4 kcalories per gram
   b. are soluble in water
   c. contain vitamins C and B_1
   d. are also known as lipids *

8. Cholesterol:
   a. is found in nuts
   b. is not produced by the body
   c. is a fat-like substance *
   d. is not found in fish and chicken

9. The requirement for unsaturated fats:
   a. is 20% of dietary kcalories *
   b. depends on one's age, height, and gender
   c. is a higher percentage for adults than for children
   d. is difficult to meet in a vegetarian diet

Match the letter of the term in Column A with the appropriate statement in Column B

A

____ 10. Fats (d)

____ 11. Cholesterol (f)

____ 12. Proteins (b)

____ 13. Essential fatty acids (c)

____ 14. Carbohydrate (a)

____ 15. Essential amino acid (e)

B

a. as sugar, it produces quick energy

b. essential for tissue building

c. must be supplied in the diet

d. spare burning of protein for energy

e. lysine

f. converted to vitamin D_3 by the action of ultraviolet light on the skin

---

16. Unsaturated fats:
    a. are found mainly in animal protein sources
    b. are usually unseen in fish *
    c. are not found in eggs
    d. none of the above

17. Saturated fats:
    a. are mainly of plant origin
    b. are liquid at cold temperatures
    c. have more hydrogen than either mono- or polyunsaturated fats *
    d. have 4 kcalories per gram

18. Sugar:
    a. should be totally avoided in meals
    b. is a form of carbohydrate *
    c. in excess is the main cause of diabetes
    d. substitutes are unsafe in moderate amounts

19. Two cups of milk, 2 ounces of meat, three vegetables, and two slices of bread supply:
    a. 10% of total kcalories in the form of protein
    b. more than 25% of the total kcalories in the form of protein
    c. 15% of total kcalories in the form of protein *
    d. 20% of total kcalories in the form of protein

20. The health care professional can help reeducate the public by:
    a. using scare tactics
    b. emphasizing about 100 g of protein in the diet
    c. promoting low fat and skim milk products and meat alternatives *
    d. arguing with the patient about health beliefs

21. A healthy meal pattern includes:
    a. 6–11 servings of bread and grains *
    b. 3 meals a day only
    c. 50 g of carbohydrate daily
    d. no fats

Match the appropriate word or words in Column B with the term in Column A

	A		**B**
____	22. macronutrients (e)	a.	gums and pectins
____	23. insoluble fiber (d)	b.	condition in which an individual lacks adequate protein
____	24. soluble fiber (a)	c.	condition in which a person lacks protein and kcalories
____	25. kwashiorkor (b)	d.	roughage
____	26. marasmus (PEM) (c)	e.	carbohydrate, protein, and fat

27. Dietary fiber:
    a. promotes dental caries
    b. is not digestible *
    c. raises blood sugar levels
    d. in the soluble form, raises cholesterol levels

28. The difference in degree of saturation relates to:
    a. the amount of fat in a food
    b. trans fatty acids in vegetable oils
    c. the amount of hydrogen in the fat molecule *
    d. the number of carbon molecules in the macronutrients

29. Triglycerides consist of:
    a. a base of glycerol and three fatty acids *
    b. water and two units of glycol
    c. two fatty acids and one molecule of oxygen
    d. carbohydrate and two glycerol units

INSTRUCTIONAL POINTS ON "A FAMILY'S PERSPECTIVE ON NUTRITION"

- Have students try to describe the food items on Maria Bernardo's shopping list. (*grain / pasta products*: italian bread, cornmeal, tagliatelle, fusilli, bucatini, and pastini; *milk products*: mozzarella and ricotta; *legumes*: chickpeas, fava beans, cannelini beans; *meat and meat substitutes*: anchovies, anchovy paste, tuna, pignoli nuts; *fats*: olive oil, unsalted butter; *vegetables*: canned tomatoes, frozen vegetables, fresh carrots; *fruits*: oranges and dried fruits; *miscellaneous / free*: balsamic vinegar, capers, garlic, basil).

- Have any of the students heard of all of these Italian foods? How many have used olive oil, or tried chickpeas, pignoli nuts (pine nuts) or capers? Could students find fava beans or cannelini beans in local grocery stores? Have students consider the impact of food choices available in grocery stores on typical U.S. eating habits. Can any of the students discuss food choices in other countries where they may have lived or in various regions of the United States?

- Have students discuss the impact of common American snack foods (ice cream, soda, baked goods, and chips) on our health. Are these snack foods that we would want other countries of the world to adopt?

ANSWERS TO TEXTBOOK STUDY QUESTIONS AND ACTIVITIES

1. Simple sugars (monosaccharides and disaccharides), complex carbohydrates, and dietary fiber (both polysaccharides).

2. Contributes to the development of dental caries; may replace other important foods in the diet; often found in high-fat foods, which contribute to the development of obestiy.

3. Soluble fiber dissolves in water and is found in high amounts in legumes, oat products, barley, brown rice, citrus fruit, the white part of the apple, and many vegetables

Insoluble fiber does not dissolve in water and is found in high amounts in the skins and seeds of vegetables and fruits, and whole wheat products

4. Legumes—lentils, chickpeas (garbanzo beans or ceci beans in Italy), fava beans, black-eyed peas, cannelini beans, kidney beans, lima beans, baked beans (navy beans)

5.

Breakfast	**Lunch**
2 oz whole grain cereal (4 g fiber)	salad w/ 1/4 cup chickpeas (5 g fiber)
milk (0 g fiber)	1/2 c. lentil soup (10 g)
orange (2 g fiber)	milk (0 g fiber)
d'caf coffee (0 g fiber)	

Supper

pasta w/ olive oil and
   anchovies (1 g fiber) and
   1/4 c. fava beans (5 g)
1/2 c. vegetables (2 g)
1 oz. cheese (0 g fiber)
   with 1/4 dried fruit (2 g)

6. Low-saturated fat foods on Maria's shopping list include: pasta, legumes, anchovies, tuna, olive oil, vinegar, capers, pignoli nuts, tomatoes, spices, vegetables, bran cereal

7. Proteins differ from carbohydrates and fats in that they contain nitrogen, which gives protein its unique function of building and repairing body tissues.

8. A complete protein contains all of the essential amino acids, which the incomplete protein sources do not (milk and milk products, red meat, fish, chicken, and eggs all contain complete protein).

9. Overconsumption of protein may lead to nutritional problems such as obesity and a calcium imbalance. Protein-energy mal-nutrition, or marasmus, and kwashiorkor are two severe nutritional problems associated with too little protein in the diet. A moderate protein deficiency can result in muscle loss, which is more likely to occur with weight-loss attempts and in the elderly.

10. The minimum number of servings adds up to just under 1200 kcalories (1178) by using 6 bread, 3 vegetables, 2 fruits, 2 cups (2%) milk, and 4 ounces of average fat content meat. There is 159 g carbohydrate (54 % of kcalories), 68 g protein (23 % of kcalories) and 30 g fat (23 % of kcalories). (Added fats and sugars are not counted.)

The maximum number of servings adds up to just under 2,000 kcalories (1985) by using 11 bread, 5 vegetables, 4 fruits, 3 cups (2 %) milk, and 6 ounces of average fat content meat (6 ounces is usually the recommended maximum intake of meat per day). This provides 286 g carbohydrate (58 % of kcalories), 109 g protein (22 % of kcalories), and 45 g fat (20 % of kcalories). (Added fats and sugars are not counted.)

11. Example: If the label reads for four crackers: 10 g carbohydrate and 5 g of fat, then six crackers would equal 15 g carbohydrate (equal to the amount of a slice of bread and should equate approximately with the size of a slice of bread) and 8 g of fat.

12. If the bagel contains 60 g carbohydrate this is equivalent to 4 slices of bread and the bagel would weigh 4 ounces (15 g carbohydrate per 1 oz slice of bread).

AUDIOVISUAL AIDS AND SUGGESTED READING

NUTRITION. This 6:40-minute videotape examines the most common nutrients, how they make up the basic food groups, and how our bodies process them. Price: $45.00. Available from NASCO, 901 Janesville Ave., Fort Atkinson, Wisconsin 53538-0901 or call 1-800-558-9595 or fax 414-563-8296.

SUPERMARKET SAVVY® TOUR VIDEO. A 52-minute videotape that takes you on an aisle-by-aisle tour of a grocery store with a registered dietitian. Emphasis is on choosing food products containing the most nutrients for the fewest calories (in relation to the carbohydrate, protein, and fat content—the energy nutrients). Price: $49.95. Available from NASCO (use above ordering information).

DIGESTION, ABSORPTION, AND METABOLISM: FOOD FOR GROWTH AND REPAIR

CHAPTER

4

SAMPLE TEST QUESTIONS

1. The term digestibility of food refers to:
    a. the amount of carbohydrate, protein, and fat in the diet
    b. the volume of food eaten at a meal
    c. the rapidity and ease of digestion as well as to its completeness *
    d. where the food is broken down in the gastrointestinal tract

2. Digestion of carbohydrates is begun in the:
    a. stomach
    b. mouth *
    c. small intestine
    d. pancreas

3. Food is changed into a semi-liquid state in the stomach and is called:
    a. starch
    b. chyme *
    c. amylase
    d. dextrin

4. Hydrochloric acid is found in the:
    a. gallbladder
    b. small intestine
    c. stomach *
    d. esophagus

5. Water is absorbed in the:
    a. large intestine *
    b. small intestine
    c. stomach
    d. pancreas

6. The end product of protein digestion is:
    a. glucose
    b. lactose
    c. dextrin
    d. amino acids *

7. Rhythmic movements that propel food through the digestive tract are called:
    a. hydrolysis
    b. peristalsis *
    c. circulation
    d. metabolism

Match the letter of the phrase in Column B with the appropriate term in Column A

A	**B**
____ 8. mouth (d)	a. forms chyme
____ 9. esophagus (e)	b. rids body of waste materials
____ 10. small intestine (c)	c. completes carbohydrate digestion
____ 11. large intestine (b)	d. generates saliva
____ 12. stomach (a)	e. joins mouth to stomach

Match the letter of the function in Column B with the appropriate hormone in Column A

A	**B**
____ 13. adrenaline (f)	a. helps regulate lipid metabolism
____ 14. cortisol (e)	b. inhibits the effect of insulin
____ 15. thyroxine (a)	c. produced by the pituitary gland
____ 16. estrogen (b)	d. facilitates the entry of blood glucose into the cells
____ 17. growth hormone (c)	e. produced in increased amounts during sleep and works opposite of insulin
____ 18. insulin (d)	f. may raise the blood sugar if there is insufficient insulin

19. Dietary fiber:
    a. is broken down by enzymes
    b. is indigestible *
    c. is found in all foods
    d. is necessary for food to move through the intestines

20. In the Krebs cycle:
    a. metabolic reactions occur when the body needs energy *
    b. vitamins are broken down for energy
    c. weight fluctuations occur
    d. amino acids are converted to fat

21. In the stomach:
    a. hydrochloric acid hinders the solubility of calcium and iron
    b. milk protein is coagulated by pepsin and partially digested by renin
    c. emulsified fats are digested to fatty acids and glycerol by lipase *
    d. mucus reduces food to a semi liquid state

Match the definition in Column B with the term in Column A

A	**B**
____ 22. glycogen (g)	a. energy supplied by the stimulating effect of food
____ 23. basal metabolism (c)	b. middle section of the small intestine
____ 24. villi (h)	c. amount of energy required for body processes
____ 25. jejunum (b)	d. lower section of the small intestine
____ 26. hydrolysis (f)	e. of a constructive nature
____ 27. specific dynamic action (a)	f. involves the addition of water to molecules
____ 28. ileum (d)	g. sugar stored in the liver
____ 29. anabolism (e)	h. finger-like projections in the intestines

---

30. Absorption:
    a. takes place mostly in the large intestine
    b. is a process that allows materials to be carried by the blood to various organs and tissues *
    c. takes place mainly in the mouth
    d. is the passage of soluble digested food materials through arterial walls

31. In the case study mini series, Tony Bernardo:
    a. has lactose intolerance
    b. was learning how balanced meals could slow the digestion of food *
    c. would be able to eat as much as he desired
    d. had no risk factors for heart disease

32. Basal metabolic rate is influenced by:
    a. gender, body size, and age
    b. body composition, height, and weight
    c. body composition, body size, and age *
    d. total energy requirement of the individual

33. Basal metabolic rate is estimated by:
    a. multiplying one's weight in pounds by .9 for a woman and by 1.0 for a man and then by 24
    b. multiplying one's weight in kilograms by .9 for a woman and by 1.0 for a man and then by 24 *
    c. adding one's weight in pounds and then multiplying by 24
    d. none of the above

34. Protein, carbohydrate, and fat digestion are completed in the small intestine.
    a. true *
    b. false

35. Fatty foods take longer to digest than fruits, vegetables, bread, and meat.
    a. true *
    b. false

36. Mucus in the stomach protects the lining of the stomach from hydrochloric acid.
    a. true *
    b. false

INSTRUCTIONAL POINTS ON "A FAMILY'S PERSPECTIVE ON NUTRITION"

- Can students describe how their own hunger is better controlled with balanced meals versus for example a donut and coffee for breakfast? Do any of the students watch fat or sugar grams on food labels?
- Have students describe their personal strategies to control stress.

ANSWERS TO TEXTBOOK STUDY QUESTIONS

1. The purpose of digestion is to change food from complex to simpler forms and from an insoluble to a soluble state in the digestive tract so as to facilitate absorption through intestinal walls into the circulation for eventual use by the body.

2. Absorption is the passage of soluble digested food materials through the intestinal walls into the blood, either directly or by way of the lymph, by means of osmosis. Absorption takes place mainly in the small intestine, lower duodenum, and upper jejunum.

3. Carbohydrates are absorbed in the form of simple sugars, fats in the form of fatty acids and glycerol, and protein in the form of amino acids.

4. Balanced meals with protein and fat will slow the digestive process of carbohydrate foods and help decrease the rate at which glucose enters the bloodstream.

5. Hormones affecting Mr. Bernardo's blood sugar levels:
   - Epinephrine (also known as adrenaline; produced in response to stress) will raise blood sugar levels
   - Cortisol and growth hormone (produced during sleep) will raise morning blood sugar levels
   - Insulin (normally excreted in response to rising blood sugar levels) will lower blood sugar levels (although the efficiency of this is reduced the form of diabetes that Mr. Bernardo has).

6. Taking baking soda for indigestion might retard stomach digestion because it reduces the acidity of the stomach, which hampers the action of digestive enzymes.

7. Energy from the Krebs cycle is made available for use by the body by breaking down the end products of digestion further. Glucose, for example (see Fig. 4–5 in the text), is broken down into pyruvate and acetyl CoA. Acetyl CoA splits and produces energy. Five percent of the fat molecule is converted to glycerol, which can yield glucose and energy also.

   NOTE: It is more important for the students to recognize that the chemical process of energy release by the body is very complex, rather than to memorize the terms of pyruvate and acetyl CoA.

8. Maltase is the enzyme that breaks down maltose; lactase breaks down lactose.

PRACTICAL APPLICATION

The student should explain that the meal of a ham sandwich, milk, and a fresh apple contains carbohydrate, protein, and fat and should be able to describe the mechanical and chemical processes as diagrammed in Figure 4–4 in the textbook.

AUDIOVISUAL AIDS AND SUGGESTED READING

EFFECTS OF MALNUTRITION ON THE BODY. Flipchart with female anatomical body systems reviewed plus overhead transparency set. Price for both: $69.99; transparency only: $24.99. Send check or money order to: Bonny Tabah, RD & Associates, 6915 E. Orange Blossom Drive, Paradise Valley, AZ 85253 or call 602-945-1797.

THE ANATOMICAL SERIES. By P. Bachin and E. Beck. An anatomical chart series that includes the digestive tract and the vascular system in a spiral notebook. Price: $54.95. Available from Health Edco, Education for Life 1993 Catalog, P.O. Box 21207, Waco, TX 76702-1207 or call 1-800-299-3366, extension 295 or fax 817-751-0221.

THE NEW NUTRITION PYRAMID. This 13-minute videotape assists the students to look at personal eating habits, analyzing diets, and the relationship between what they eat and how they exercise—their body weight, look, and composition. A systems approach is emphasized comparing the body to an engine and food to fuel. Price: $69.00. Available from NASCO, 901 Janesville Ave., Fort Atkinson, Wisconsin 53538-0901 or call 1-800-558-9595 or fax 414-563-8296.

VITAMINS, MINERALS, ELECTROLYTES, AND WATER

CHAPTER 5

SAMPLE TEST QUESTIONS

1. Vitamins:
   a. provide energy
   b. are all synthesized by the body
   c. are needed in large amounts
   d. are necessary for proper growth and development *

2. Water soluble vitamins:
   a. can be stored in the liver
   b. do not have to be included in the diet on a regular basis
   c. are found in citrus fruits *
   d. are found in margarine

3. Fat soluble vitamins:
   a. are more stable than water soluble vitamins *
   b. are found in all foods
   c. must be supplied daily
   d. cannot be stored by the body

4. The term vitamin B complex refers to:
   a. only thiamine and riboflavin
   b. only niacin and folacin
   c. all water soluble vitamins except ascorbic acid *
   d. vitamin B_6 and vitamin B_{12}

5. Vitamin C is:
   a. always toxic in high doses
   b. found in bread and cereal
   c. stored in the body
   d. involved in changing folate to folic acid *

6. Vitamin A is important in:
   a. helping eyes to adapt to dim light *
   b. the formation of hemoglobin
   c. preventing scurvy
   d. preventing rickets

7. Vitamin E is responsible for:
   a. absorption of vitamin C
   b. protecting red blood cells from rupturing *
   c. destroying vitamin A
   d. oxidizing polyunsaturated fatty acids

8. If a person has vitamin K deficiency, which of the following is likely to occur?
   a. acne
   b. formation of blood clots
   c. excessive bleeding *
   d. acidosis

9. A person who consumes the recommended amounts of milk or milk products will have an adequate intake of:
   a. vitamins D and B_2 *
   b. iron
   c. vitamin A
   d. thiamine

10. Which of the following is not a good source of vitamin A?
    a. dark green leafy vegetables
    b. orange vegetables and fruits
    c. liver
    d. whole wheat bread *

Match the letter of the term in Column B with the appropriate term in Column A

A   **B**

____ 11. Fat-soluble vitamins (c)   a. Vitamin K

____ 12. Water-soluble vitamins (f)   b. Retinol or preformed

____ 13. Toxic forms of vitamin A   c. Vitamins A, D, E, and K
              (in excess) (b)
                                                                          d. Riboflavin
____ 14. Excess causes skin to turn yellow (g)
                                                                          e. Rebound scurvy
____ 15. Obtained from sunlight (h)
                                                                          f. B complex and vitamin C
____ 16. Synthesized from bacteria in
              the intestines (a)   g. Carotene

____ 17. Easily destroyed (j)   h. Vitamin D

____ 18. Light-sensitive vitamin in milk (d)   i. Vitamin B_{12}

____ 19. Deficiency causes pernicious   j. Water-soluble vitamins
              anemia (i)

____ 20. A condition that may develop
              when megadoses of vitamin C
              are abruptly stopped (e)

---

21. Inadequate iodine intake leads to:
    a. anemia
    b. goiter *
    c. rickets
    d. osteoporosis

22. Electrolytes are responsible for:
    a. acid-base balance *
    b. blood sugar levels
    c. hemoglobin levels
    d. hormone levels

23. Which of the following are *all* good sources of
    potassium?
    a. bananas, oranges, meats *
    b. potatoes, apples, carrots
    c. cranberries, bananas, rice
    d. noodles, rice, potatoes

24. Water requirements are increased for:
    a. fever
    b. diarrhea
    c. high-fiber diets
    c. all of the above *

Match the description in Column B with the mineral in Column A

A

____ 25. calcium (f)

____ 26. potassium (b)

____ 27. sodium (j)

____ 28. sulfur (g)

____ 29. chromium (c)

____ 30. cobalt (d)

____ 31. fluorine (i)

____ 32. iron (a)

____ 33. selenium (h)

____ 34. zinc (e)

B

a. helps growth and development through its role in the formation of hemoglobin

b. transmits nerve impulses; found in high amounts in apricots, raisins, and potatoes

c. enhances the removal of glucose from blood

d. an essential component of vitamin B_{12}

e. essential for wound healing, immune function, and taste acuity

f. helps muscles to contract and relax, thereby helping to regulate heartbeat

g. part of three amino acids, vitamin B_1 and biotin

h. acts as an antioxidant with vitamin E to protect the cell from oxygen

i. recommended in supplement form for children (unless in the water supply) to prevent dental caries

j. along with potassium, plays a key role in fluid balance

35. Vitamin B_{12}:
    a. is present in large amounts in green leafy vegetables
    b. is not found in milk
    c. prevents scurvy
    d. requires a glycoprotein secreted in the stomach to aid its absorption *

36. Supplement usage may be indicated for:
    a. all babies under 6 months
    b. women with excessive menstrual bleeding *
    c. athletes
    d. teenagers who eat fast foods on a regular basis

37. Iron absorption can be improved by:
    a. drinking milk daily
    b. consuming foods high in vitamin A
    c. eating meat and foods high in vitamin C *
    d. storing food properly

38. A high-risk group for folate deficiency is:
    a. premature, low birth-weight infants *
    b. men over 65 years of age
    c. athletes
    d. persons of Chinese heritage

INSTRUCTIONAL POINTS ON "A FAMILY'S PERSPECTIVE ON NUTRITION"

- Review a periodic table for common minerals found in food. Ask students why Joey Bernardo might confuse minerals with vitamins.
- Use overhead transparency (Fig. 6–2) to show a new food label. Have students identify the macronutrients from the minerals and vitamins.

ANSWERS TO TEXTBOOK STUDY QUESTIONS AND ACTIVITIES

1. Minerals do not break down because they are elemental in nature, not being composed of several elements as vitamins are (carbon, hydrogen, oxygen, and other nutrients).

2. Foods that contain vitamins must be eaten daily to ensure adequate intake and because certain ones cannot be stored and thus are needed daily. (Fat soluble vitamins are stored; water soluble ones generally are not.)

3. The B-complex includes all water soluble vitamins except vitamin C. Whole grains, enriched bread products, legumes, milk, organ meats and other meats, and dark green, leafy vegetables supply all of the essential B vitamins.

4. Grains—6 to 11 servings
   Vegetables—3 to 5 servings
   Fruits—2 to 4 servings
   Milk—2 to 3 servings
   Meat—2 to 3 servings

   Yes, foods from Maria Bernardo's shopping list could meet the RDA for the following nutrients:
   - Cheese—protein, calcium, phosphorus, magnesium, vitamins B_2, B_{12} and D (if whole milk cheese)
   - Legumes—protein, calcium, phosphorus, magnesium, and iron
   - Frozen vegetables—vitamins A and C, potassium, phosphorus
   - Bran cereal—B complex
   - Pignoli nuts—protein, magnesium
   - Pasta—B complex and iron

5. Legume food ideas:
   - Pasta with beans
   - Salad with chickpeas
   - Lentil salad or lentil soup
   - Pasta fazula (pronounced fazule—pasta and bean soup)
   - Chili con carne
   - Bean burrito
   - Hopping John (black-eyed peas and rice)
   - Four bean salad with chickpeas
   - Succotash (lima beans with creamed corn)

6. Have students refer to the Appendix Food Composition Table for calcium content of foods. (Chapters 1 and 5 also provide common sources of calcium.)

7. Procedures in food care, preparation, and cooking that help retain water soluble vitamins:
   - Store produce to prevent wilting and drying out
   - Cook vegetables whole or in large pieces
   - Steam or microwave vegetables, avoiding overcooking
   - Use cooking water from vegetables in soups
   - Avoid using baking soda when cooking vegetables
   - Cover or refrigerate fats
   - Keep milk away from light
   - Use meat drippings (fat can be removed)
   - Cover fruit juices and keep refrigerated after opening containers
   - Avoid stirring foods containing vitamin C while they are cooking
   - Cover and refrigerate leftovers

8. Role-play situation:
   Business woman who relies on vitamin pills because she believes they are a good replacement for her poor vegetable intake (lack of knowledge), and because she does not like many vegetables (food dislikes), and does not have time to cook them (inadequate food habits).

   Possible advice:
   Lack of knowledge—Explain that there are other nutrients found in vegetables and fruits, such as fiber, not found in vitamin pills. Point out that vitamin A (not beta carotene) can be toxic and should be avoided in pill form by women of child-bearing years.

Food dislikes—Suggest vegetables in alternate forms such as spinach salad, coleslaw, vegetable soup, or tomato juice. Fruits may take the place of some vegetables, especially the deep orange ones (apricots, cantaloupe, watermelon, peaches).

Inadequate food habits (lack of time)—suggest ideas for quick meals and snacks such as dried apricots, cantaloupe wedges, extra tomato on sandwiches.

Vitamin A food ideas:

- Melt cheese onto broccoli to increase its taste appeal
- Cut orange cantaloupe into balls (using a device for this purpose) and serve with green honeydew melon for visual appeal
- Top sweet potatoes with marshmallows or honey and cinnamon for taste appeal
- Stuff a whole tomato (cut into a flower-like shape) with tuna salad or cottage cheese for a quick meal idea

- Cut carrots into curls with a vegetable peeler or shred using a grater for visual appeal
- Slice carrots on the slant for visual appeal for use in salads
- Make carrot and raisin salad with pineapple chunks for a sweet side dish
- Put chopped spinach into layers of lasagna

AUDIOVISUAL AIDS AND SUGGESTED READING

RECOMMENDED DIETARY ALLOWANCES, 10th ed., 1989. By the National Research Council. This reference presents information and insights with widespread practical application on nutrient allowances for the maintenance of good health. Price: $14.95. Available from Nutrition Counseling Education Service, 1904 E. 123rd Street, Olathe, KS 66061 or call 1-800-445-5653 or fax 913-782-8230.

GUIDES FOR GOOD FOOD CHOICES

CHAPTER 6

SAMPLE TEST QUESTIONS

1. Legumes were placed in the meat group of the Food Guide Pyramid because they are high in:
   a. carbohydrate
   b. protein *
   c. fat
   d. kcalories

2. The RDAs are:
   a. the daily requirement for an individual
   b. recommendations for the average daily amounts of nutrients that population groups should consume over a certain period *
   c. used for determining the adequacy of a diet even if it is supplemented
   d. the estimated minimum requirements of most healthy individuals

3. The new RDIs (Reference Daily Intake):
   a. are used only on nutrition labels for processed foods
   b. required on all labels of most regulated foods *
   c. were developed by the Food and Nutrition Board
   d. show the amount of food needed in one day to assure a well-balanced diet

Match terms in Column A with definitions in Column B

A	**B**
____ 4. Daily Reference Values (e)	a. recommended nutrients for populations
____ 5. Dietary Guidelines (d)	b. developed by the Food & Drug Administration for use in nutrition labeling
____ 6. RDIs (b)	
____ 7. The Food Guide Pyramid (c)	c. emphasis is on the consumption of plant foods
____ 8. RDAs (a)	
	d. seven recommendations that taken together address the relationship between diet and chronic diseases
	e. are found on the new food labels and are based on percentages of 2,000 kcalories

Match the terms in Column A with the appropriate definition in Column B

A	**B**

A

_____ 9. Moderation (a)

_____ 10. Variety (c)

_____ 11. Balance (b)

_____ 12. Allowance (d)

B

a. refers to amounts of food for a healthy body weight

b. means to choose foods with enough protein, vitamins, minerals, and fiber but not too much sodium, sugar, fat, and alcohol

c. refers to eating some foods from each of the five food groups

d. refers to the amount of nutrient that must be consumed in order to insure that the requirements of most people are met

---

13. The suggested minimum number of servings in the Food Guide Pyramid averages:
    a. about 1,500 kcalories
    b. about 2,000 kcalories
    c. about 1,200 kcalories *
    d. about 3,000 kcalories

14. The Food Guide Pyramid:
    a. is a five food group system
    b. illustrates how to meet maximum daily requirements
    c. illustrates how to meet minimum daily requirements
    d. all of the above *

15. The U.S. Dietary Guidelines are:
    a. Eat a variety of foods
    b. Maintain a healthy weight
    c. Choose foods low in fat, saturated fat, and cholesterol
    d. Choose a diet with plenty of grain products, vegetables, and fruits
    e. Use sugars only in moderation
    f. Use salt and sodium only in moderation
    g. If you drink alcoholic beverages, do so in moderation

16. The Food Guide Pyramid recommends the following number of servings each day:
    Breads and cereals —6 to 11
    Fruits —2 to 4
    Vegetables —3 to 5
    Meat, poultry, fish, eggs, legumes, nuts and peanut butter —2 to 3
    Milk, yogurt, and cheese —2 to 3

17. Daily Reference Values for fat, saturated fat, carbohydrate, protein, and fiber are expressed in percentages of total kcalories or grams as follows:
    Fat — 30%
    Saturated fat—10%
    Carbohydrate — 60%
    Protein —10%
    Fiber — 25 g

18. According to the Food Guide Pyramid the following serving sizes are recommended:
    cooked cereal or pasta —1 ounce or 1/2 cup
    fruit juice — 3/4 cup
    cooked vegetables —1/2 cup
    raw vegetables or salad —1 cup
    meat — 2–3 ounces
    peanut butter — 2 Tbsp
    milk —1 cup

19. Following the U.S. Dietary Guidelines will guarantee health and well-being.
    a. true
    b. false *

20. The reference for sodium intake on the new food label is:
    a. 500 mg per day
    b. 1,000 mg per day
    c. 2,400 mg per day *
    d. 3,000 mg per day

21. The incidence of chronic and degenerative diseases is primarily the result of:
    a. dietary excesses and imbalances *
    b. a lack of exercise
    c. eating 12 servings of breads and grain products daily
    d. not taking vitamin supplements

22. The age to which the allowance of 1,200 mg calcium has been extended to is:
    a. 51 years
    b. 75 years
    c. 25 years *
    d. 30 years

23. The iron allowance in the RDAs for women through age 50 is now:
    a. 18 mg
    b. 15 mg *
    c. 10 mg
    d. 20 mg

24. It is almost impossible to take in toxic amounts of vitamin A by eating broccoli and carrots daily.
    a. true *
    b. false

25. The RDAs are more complex and technical than the Dietary Guidelines for Americans.
    a. true *
    b. false

26. Children instinctively know how to make food choices to stay healthy.
    a. true
    b. false *

27. It is easy to meet nutritional needs by only including plant foods in the diet
    a. true
    b. false *

INSTRUCTIONAL POINTS ON "A FAMILY'S PERSPECTIVE ON NUTRITION"

- Ask students if any of them had known the Food Guide Pyramid can help with weight control and heart disease.
- Discuss ways people learn about food and health management such as in health class or from a registered dietitian. Do any of the students read journal articles or books on improving their health through wise food choices?

ANSWERS TO TEXTBOOK STUDY QUESTIONS AND ACTIVITIES

1. The Dietary Guidelines for Americans are general and unstructured. The Food Guide Pyramid provides recommended servings and portions to meet health needs. By aiming to have the base of the diet as whole grains, and the tip of the diet or least amount of food in the diet as added fats and sugars, as portrayed in the Pyramid, the Dietary Guidelines for less fat and sugar and more fiber can be met. Avoiding added salt will further help meet the Dietary Guidelines.

2. The RDAs should not be used to evaluate an individual's diet because specific requirements for individuals may vary and are ordinarily unknown. Certain medical problems such as infections and chronic disease affect nutrient needs.

3. Factors that affect an individual's nutrient requirements include premature birth, inherited metabolic disorders, infections, chronic disease, and the use of medications

4. The RDAs are meant to serve as a general guide for evaluating and planning adequate diets for healthy population groups.

5. Students should indicate in red pencil the requirement for kcalories and all nutrients for a person of their age.

6. Students should bring to class some sample nutrition labels and show how to use the percentage values in planning a day's menu. For example to provide 100 % of the daily need for calcium the percentages found on food labels should add up to a total of about 100 % for calcium.

7. Grain group: cornmeal, pastas: tagliatelle, fusilli, bucatini, and pastini, bran cereal (flour probably found in the home)
   Vegetable group: canned tomatoes, frozen vegetables
   Fruit group: (none listed on her shopping list)

Milk group: mozzarella and ricotta cheese (milk probably found in the home due to their eating cereal)

Meat group: lentils, chickpeas, fava and cannelini beans, pancetta, anchovies and anchovy paste, tuna, and pignoli nuts.

Note: Capers are not likely to provide any significant nutritional value as they are used as a condiment only. They are the unopened flowers of the caper bush, a shrub native to the Mediterranean region and are preserved in vinegar and salt. Garlic generally does not provide any significant nutritional value due to small portions consumed, although in significant quantities (three or more garlic cloves per day) may have a health impact.

---

8. A menu using the maximum number of food servings from the Food Guide Pyramid (about 2,000 kcalories not counting added fats and assuming cheese and milk are low fat) from Maria's shopping list with assumed fruits and milk found in the Bernardo home:

BREAKFAST	LUNCH	SUPPER
2 oz bran cereal with 1 c. milk medium banana 2 oz ricotta cheese	2 large slices pizza w/ 1 1/2 oz mozzarella 2 c. salad with 1/2 c. chickpeas and 3 oz tuna and oil/vinegar dressing 1/2 c. pineapple slices for dessert 6 oz fruit juice	2 c. pasta (4 oz) with 1/2 c. beans lightly seasoned with olive oil, capers, garlic and pignoli nuts and 1 oz anchovy 1/2 cup polenta 1 1/2 cups cooked vegetables 1 medium apple

---

9. Anna Bernardo's menu can be analyzed according to the Food Guide Pyramid as follows:

banana—1 fruit

corn flakes (each ounce equals 1 bread group serving)

whole milk (1 cup equals 1 milk serving)

toast (one slice equals 1 bread serving)

hot dog (equals 1 oz meat for average size hot dog)

hot dog roll (2 bread servings)

chocolate chip cookies (2 small equals about 1 bread serving)

cheeseburger (average size about 3 oz meat; 1 slice cheese equals 1/2 milk serving)

hamburger roll (2 bread servings)

french fries (1 small order equals 1 serving vegetable)

coleslaw (1 scoop equals 1 serving vegetable)

milkshake (12 oz size equals 1 1/2 milk servings)

According to the minimum number of recommended servings of the Food Guide Pyramid, this menu meets the grain servings (although whole grain rolls and bread would be recommended), the vegetable and fruit groups are both lacking one serving each (and a high vitamin A source should be included), there are three servings of milk consumed (which will provide just under 1,000 mg calcium — a bit low for Anna with the RDA being 1,200 mg), 4 oz meat meets the minimum recommended amount of meat servings.

The foods and amounts lacking in Anna's diet:
- 1 c. of milk should be added to meet the RDA (even thought the Pyramid sets the servings at three maximum)
- 1/2 c. dark green leafy vegetable should be added for folate

- 1 c. cantaloupe would provide the extra serving of fruit while providing vitamin A (beta-carotene) and vitamin C

Anna is not likely to lose weight with this menu due to the high fat content. She would be better off eating a baked potato versus french fries, a tossed salad versus coleslaw, low-fat milk versus a milkshake and for her cereal, to use added butter, jelly, and sugar sparingly, a turkey sandwich versus a hot dog, and a hamburger versus a cheeseburger (unless it is low-fat cheese; low-fat milk to drink can better provide calcium), and to eat fruit for dessert versus high fat cookies. She might try diet soda or water in place of the coke to drink.

AUDIOVISUAL AIDS AND SUGGESTED READING

THE FOOD GUIDE PYRAMID: CONTEMPORARY NUTRITION. A 30-minute videotape that highlights the foods from the major food groups and their relationship to the Dietary Guidelines for Americans. Price: $79.95. Available from NASCO, 901 Janesville Ave., Fort Atkinson, Wisconsin 53538-0901 or call 1-800-558-9595 or fax 414-563-8296.

UNDERSTANDING FOOD LABELS. A comprehensive brochure for consumer education. Price: $4.89 ($4.00 ADA members). Available from The American Dietetic Association, 216 W. Jackson Blvd., Chicago, IL 60606-6995 or call 312-899-0040.

NUTRITION IN THE INSTITUTIONAL SETTING: THE INTERPLAY BETWEEN CHRONIC AND ACUTE ILLNESS

CHAPTER 7

SAMPLE TEST QUESTIONS

Match the definition in Column B with the appropriate term in Column A. Answers may be used more than once.

A

_____ 1. Addison's disease (c)

_____ 2. Gout (e)

_____ 3. Osteomalacia (a)

_____ 4. Polyneuritis (b)

_____ 5. Uremia (d)

_____ 6. Wilson's disease (c)

B

a. a condition in which the bones become soft

b. inflammation of the nerves

c. a disease in which the body stores excess amounts of copper

d. an excess in the blood of nitrogenous end products of protein metabolism

e. a disease of the joints

---

7. A diet is termed qualitative when the adaptations are:
   a. in types of food or consistency *
   b. increases or decreases of certain nutrients or kcalories
   c. changes in temperature of food
   d. when the meals are served

8. Patients with reactive hypoglycemia need a diet that provides:
   a. meals with little or no protein at each meal
   b. six small meals *
   c. concentrated sweets
   d. 10-15 g of fat at each meal

9. A ketongenic diet is needed to control:
   a. weight
   b. diabetes
   c. a type of epilepsy *
   d. uremia

10. A fat controlled low cholesterol diet is used for individuals with:
    a. atherosclerosis *
    b. high triglycerides
    c. seizures
    d. phenylketonuria

11. A restrictive protein diet is used for patients with:
    a. cardiovascular disease
    b. chronic uremia *
    c. lactose intolerance
    d. dumping syndrome

12. A modified carbohydrate diet is used for individuals with:
    a. increased metabolism
    b. pernicious anemia
    c. lactose intolerance *
    d. Addison's disease

13. An increased sodium diet is useful in:
    a. Addison's disease *
    b. congestive heart failure
    c. hypertension
    d. diverticulosis

14. Shellfish, liver, legumes, and whole grains all contain _____ , which should be restricted in Wilson's disease.
    a. calcium
    b. B vitamins
    c. copper *
    d. protein

15. Anemia, which is treated with high-iron foods and vitamin C, is:
    a. pernicious anemia
    b. megaloblastic anemia
    c. iron-deficiency anemia *
    d. all of the above

16. Individuals with celiac disease require:
    a. a restricted protein diet
    b. a low-tyramine diet
    c. a gluten-free diet *
    d. a high-protein diet

17. A restricted purine diet is useful in treating:
    a. hepatic coma
    b. gout *
    c. renal disease
    d. tropical sprue

18. Pernicious anemia is treated with a diet high in:
    a. protein *
    b. sodium
    c. iron
    d. vitamin C

19. Tetany is related to low blood levels of:
    a. iron
    b. hemoglobin
    c. glucose
    d. calcium *

20. Night blindness requires a diet high in:
    a. vitamin C
    b. vitamin E
    c. vitamin A *
    d. vitamin K

21. Cystic fibrosis and malabsorption syndromes are diagnosed by a:
    a. glucose tolerance test
    b. meat-free test diet
    c. calcium test
    d. fecal fat determination diet *

22. In the custodial approach of long-term care:
    a. patients would be fed by the staff *
    b. patients would be encouraged to self-feed with assistance only by the staff
    c. patients would be encouraged to walk or wheelchair to the dining area
    d. patients would be allowed to do things for themselves

23. Triceps skin folds is:
    a. an index of the level of the body's protein stores
    b. an indicator of body frame size
    c. is an index of the body's fat or energy stores *
    d. used for only men

24. Mid arm circumference:
    a. is an index of the body's fat or energy stores
    b. indicates the level of the body's protein stores *
    c. is easy to measure on obese people
    d. a measurement of body frame size

25. Diuretics:
    a. bind with enzymes and affect the metabolism of some nutrients
    b. may result in weight gain
    c. can be potassium depleting *
    d. have an effect on appetite

INSTRUCTIONAL POINTS ON "A FAMILY'S PERSPECTIVE ON NUTRITION"

- Have students discuss how a disruption in family routine, such as the hospitalization of a mother, impacts on family food choices and eating habits.
- Do any of the students know of anyone who had severe morning sickness or hyperemesis of pregnancy?
- Can the students imagine how it would feel for a pregnant woman with hyperemesis to hear babies crying in the hospital?
- Have any of the students been hospitalized? How did it feel having to wait for meal trays to come? How was appetite affected in the hospital setting?

ANSWERS TO TEXTBOOK STUDY QUESTIONS AND ACTIVITIES

1. Six ways to modify the basic normal diet for therapeutic purposes:
   - Increase or decrease energy value.
   - Increase or decrease fiber.
   - Increase or decrease specific nutrients.
   - Increase or decrease specific foods or types of foods.
   - Alter any one of above diets to become a soft or liquid diet.
   - Eliminate condiments and any specific foods not tolerated.

2. Six considerations to remember in meal service are:
   - Food portions should be of appropriate size and attractively arranged.
   - Hot foods should be served hot; cold foods served cold.
   - Ensure pleasant meatime conversation.
   - Allow plenty of time for eating.
   - Ensure that the patient's name is on the diet ticket and that the tray is complete before serving.
   - Avoid spoiled foods or liquids.

   NOTE: These considerations are just a few of those noted in the text.

   Nurse discussions with Mrs. Bernardo should focus on positive or neutral topics such as the weather, gifts from friends, or enthusiam displayed over foods served on the tray. Nega-

tive topics should be avoided such as bad points of the meal, or emotional topics such as risks to the baby from vomiting and weight loss.

3. Possible family effects from Maria's hospital admission:
   - Eating "on the run" to visit her after school or work
   - Choosing high fat and high sodium convenience foods
   - Stress-related eating due to concerns of Maria and the baby

4. Characteristics of good nutritional status:
   - Shiny hair
   - Bright eyes
   - Flat abdomen
   - Normal weight for height, age, and body build
   - Well-developed and firm muscles
   - Good appetite and digestion

   Characteristics of poor nutritional status
   - Dull hair
   - Swollen gums
   - Missing teeth
   - Dry skin
   - Swollen abdomen

5. Food and drug interactions should be considered in the assessment process because drugs can affect nutrient absorption, excretion, and metabolism. Food as well as specific nutrients can adversely affect drug action. Interactions between food and drugs therefore can affect a person's nutritional status.

6. The assessment form on Maria Bernardo can only partially be completed due to lack of data. Have students complete this form as fully as they can and have them discuss in class where they could determine the missing pieces of information (discussions with Maria, patient chart, observation of meal tray, and so on).

   The dietitian would assess Maria Bernardo's nutritional needs and implements a nutritional care plan with the support of the physician, nurse, pharmacist, social worker, and therapists. Each of these health professionals will have input on ways to achieve goals decided on by the health care team. The completed nutritional assessment should be discussed with this in mind.

7. Appropriate reasons to consult a dietitian include the following:
   - Weight loss especially if significant (> 5%–10 % of body weight)
   - Food allergies or intolerances
   - Low serum albumin
   - Clear liquid for more than 3 days, especially if after surgery
   - Hyperlipidemia, hyperglycemia, hypertension, or hyperkalemia

8. Percentage of weight change would be calculated as follows:

$$\frac{130\ lb - 110\ lb}{130\ lb} \times 100 = \frac{20\ lb}{130\ lb} \times 100 = 15\%$$

9. A 5'10" male with an elbow breadth of 2.5 inches equals a small frame (see Appendix of text)

10. Protein calorie malnutrition (or protein energy malnutrition) can be detected in a hospital patient by monitoring the blood serum levels of albumin, transferrin, and lymphocytes, all of which are associated with body protein stores. Anthropometric measures can also help in detection.

11. A low protein diet affects primarily the meat and milk group of the Food Guide Pyramid. Grain products need to be eaten in moderate amounts. Fruits, fats, and sugars may be used for kcalorie sources as appropriate to the person's diagnosis and lab values. Using the servings of the Food Guide Pyramid the following advice may be given without jeopardizing the person's health (about 75 g protein total; a person needing less protein should consult with a dietitian):
    - 4 ounces meat or meat substitute (28 g protein)
    - 2 cups milk or yogurt (16 g protein)
    - 8 servings grains (24 g protein)
    - 5 or more servings vegetables and fruits (7 g protein)
    - added fats and sugars as appropriate

AUDIOVISUAL AIDS AND SUGGESTED READING

1992 CRITERIA OF NUTRITIONAL CARE BY DIAGNOSIS. Designed for acute care hospitals and skilled nursing facilities. Manual features patient care guidelines, methods of evaluation of weight change, nutritional assessment, intervention and outcome with suggested documentation. Price: $25.00 + $3.25 S/H (California residents add 8.25 % tax). Available from Food and Nutrition Services, Inc., 6151 W. Century Blvd., Suite 916, Los Angeles, CA 90045 or call 310-215-0352 or fax 310-215-9204.

MANUAL OF CLINICAL DIETETICS, 4th ed, 1992. Prepared by the Chicago Dietetic Association and the South Suburban Dietetic Association; covers all aspects of nutrition management during health and disease throughout the life cycle. Price: $62.00 ($52.00 ADA members). Available from The American Dietetic Association, 216 W. Jackson Blvd., Chicago, IL 60606-6995 or call 312/899-0040.

PATIENT EDUCATION MATERIALS AND INSTRUCTOR'S GUIDE: A SUPPLEMENT TO THE MANUAL OF CLINICAL DIETETICS. By J.E. Shield and M.C. Mullen. Provides two-sided reproducible masters for patient education materials on 14 of the more frequently used therapeutic diets. Price: $15.00 ($12.75 ADA members). Available from The American Dietetic Association, 216 W. Jackson Blvd., Chicago, IL 60606-6995 or call 312/899-0040.

QUANTITY FOOD PREPARATION: STANDARDIZING RECIPES AND CONTROLLING INGREDIENTS, 3rd ed. By P. Buchanan. This educational tool is useful for developing and implementing a recipe standardization program; provides detailed instructions for designing recipe format and adjusting recipe yields. Price: $18.00 ($15.00 ADA members). Available from The American Dietetic Association, 216 W. Jackson Blvd., Chicago, IL 60606-6995 or call 312/899-0040.

CHAPTER 8

CARDIOVASCULAR DISEASE

SAMPLE TEST QUESTIONS

Match the terms in Column A with the description in Column B

A

_____ 1. arteriosclerosis (d)

_____ 2. antioxidants (e)

_____ 3. hypertension (a)

_____ 4. hyperlipidemia (c)

_____ 5. edema (b)

B

a. high blood pressure

b. condition of fluid build-up

c. elevation of specific lipoproteins

d. hardening of the arteries

e. may help to prevent plaque build-up on artery walls

6. A restricted sodium diet is indicated for:
   a. cortisone therapy *
   b. elevated serum triglycerides
   c. coronary thrombosis
   d. elevated blood glucose

7. The National Cholesterol Education Program defines high risk as:
   a. cholesterol levels between 200 and 239 mg/dl
   b. cholesterol levels above 240 mg/dl *
   c. cholesterol levels above 300 mg/dl
   d. cholesterol levels below 200 mg/dl

8. Saturated fats are:
   a. found in solid animal fats
   b. found in coconut and palm oil
   c. are formed through the process of hydrogenation
   d. all of the above *

9. The form of lipoprotein that is high in triglycerides is called:
   a. HDL
   b. LDL
   c. VLDL *
   d. none of the above

10. The percentage of Americans with serum cholesterol levels over 240 mg/dl is:
    a. 10 percent
    b. 20 percent *
    c. 50 percent
    d. 75 percent

11. The medical term for stroke is:
    a. cardiovascular disease
    b. congestive heart failure
    c. coronary thrombosis
    d. cerebrovascular accident *

12. Weight loss often results in:
    a. a lowering of blood pressure
    b. a reduced incidence of coronary disease
    c. a lowering of blood lipids
    d. all of the above *

13. A fat intake of less than ____ of total kcalories can help reverse the plaquing process:
    a. 50 %
    b. 40 %
    c. 30 %
    d. 10 % *

14. The guidelines of the American Heart Association recommends:
    a. no more than 30 % of total kcalories in the form of fat *
    b. cholesterol intake no more than 200 mg per day
    c. a sodium intake of 6,000 mg per day
    d. a saturated fat intake of less than 20 % of total kcalories

15. If a fat is soft or liquid at cold temperatures it is high in:
    a. saturated fat
    b. unsaturated fats *
    c. cholesterol
    d. none of the above

16. The intake of dietary cholesterol:
    a. has a significant impact on the body's own natural cholesterol production
    b. has little impact on the body's own natural cholesterol production *
    c. is more important than reducing saturated fat intake in the diet
    d. is greatly reduced by eating fish and chicken

17. Foods that may help lower the body's own natural cholesterol production include:
    a. oatmeal, legumes, and vegetables
    b. olive oil and peanut oil
    c. walnuts
    d. all of the above *

18. Children over this age can safely reduce their fat intake to the AHA guidelines:
    a. 9 months
    b. 12 months
    c. 18 months
    d. 24 months *

19. Risk factors for cardiovascular disease include:
    a. hypertension
    b. female gender over 55 years or with premature menopause not on estrogen
    c. diabetes mellitus
    d. all of the above *

20. The National Cholesterol Education Program (NCEP) advises an LDL level of no more than:
    a. 300 mg/dl
    b. 200 mg/dl
    c. 160 mg/dl *
    d. 100 mg/dl

21. Cholesterol is found in:
    a. peanut butter
    b. chicken *
    c. coconut oil
    d. avocados

22. You can tell that eggs are low in saturated fat because:
    a. eggs do not contain cholesterol
    b. eggs are not meat
    c. eggs are liquid even at cold temperatures *
    d. none of the above

23. Persons with elevated triglyceride levels should be advised to:
    a. eat more cold water fish such as salmon *
    b. take fish oil capsules
    c. eat more catfish
    d. eat more trout

24. High sources of soluble fiber include:
    a. whole grain oat products
    b. chickpeas and lentils
    c. barley
    d. all of the above *

INSTRUCTIONAL POINTS ON "A FAMILY'S PERSPECTIVE ON NUTRITION"

Have any of the students ever had lab work after fasting all night? How did they feel about this experience?

Ask students if they know the difference between good cholesterol and bad cholesterol and have them try to describe the difference (at the end of the class study on this topic you may want to ask this question again).

ANSWERS TO TEXTBOOK STUDY QUESTIONS AND ACTIVITIES

1. Mr. Bernardo's known cardiovascular risk factors include (refer also to case study of Chapter 2):
   * Elevated cholesterol
   * Middle aged (technically over 45 years of age; date of birth not known)
   * Hypertension
   * Cigarette smoking
   * Diabetes mellitus

2. Have students interview their parents or other family members if possible to identify their personal health risk of cardiovascular disease and hypertension. (Students should be prompted to ask specific questions in reference to heart attacks and stroke versus "heart disease.")

3. Coconut oil can be found in larger grocery stores. If it cannot be found note to the class that it becomes solid at cold temperatures (a saturated fat). Use at least olive oil (which will turn viscous in the refrigerator—a monounsaturated fat) and corn oil (which will remain unchanged at cold temperatures—a polyunsaturated fat.)

4. Look for low-sodium bread, low-sodium cheese, low-sodium crackers and low-sodium tomato juice. Jelly will enhance the flavor of grain products; lemon will add flavor to tomato juice. Herbs such as basil sprinkled on the cheese or added garlic can be tasty.

5. Have students brainstorm in class a list of everyday foods and have them bring in food labels from home or from the college cafeteria for comparison. NOTE: If comparing fat contents, use a common reference such as fat per 15 g of carbohydrate (1 bread serving) or fat per 7 g of protein (1 ounce of meat).

6. Students should take a 24-hour diet history from one family member or friend with portions identified as close as possible. Sodium content can be found in the food composition table of the Appendix.

7. The health care professional in the role-play with "Mr. Bernardo" can point out that hard fats (at cold temperatures) will tend to raise the body's blood cholesterol level while soft or liquid oils will do the opposite.

   Assessment questions to ask of Mr. Bernardo include:
   * "How do you feel about using less butter and using olive oil to lower your risk of heart disease?"
   * "Do you think you are likely to change to 1 % milk and low-fat cheeses?"
   * "Can you limit anchovies to 1 oz per day to help keep sodium intake low?"
   * "If potato chips are in the house for the children can you avoid eating them?"

8. Lunch time low-fat food ideas appropriate to a construction site (suggestions listed have less than 10–15 g of fat and do not require refrigeration by noontime):
   * Sandwich with 1 Tbsp peanut butter
   * 2 oz low-fat cheese with low-fat crackers
   * 1/8 cup nuts with dried fruit and tomato sandwich with mustard
   * 2 oz lean meat sandwich (prefrozen, which will thaw by noon)

   Dessert ideas (low-fat appropriate for no refrigeration)
   * Graham crackers
   * Ginger snaps
   * Fig newtons
   * Fruit, fresh or dried

9. Have students bring favorite recipes to class. They should add up the total saturated fat and sodium per recipe (the food composition table in their textbook appendix provides this information). These totals are then divided by the desired serving size to determine the amount per serving. The goal is to have the saturated fat content less than 5 g per meal or less than 1 g per snack with sodium less than 800 mg per entree/meal and snacks less than 200 mg sodium. Have students modify recipes for reduced portions, reduced total fat use (such as replacing oil with applesauce in baked goods), change to liquid oils (lower in saturated fat), and/or reduced salt use to meet these guidelines. Students may want to prepare their modified recipe and report on its acceptance to the class.

10. Advice appropriate to provide to Mr. Bernardo to help his family prevent the development of cardiovascular disease:

- Use the concept of the Food Guide Pyramid (have plant foods as the base of the diet including pasta, vegetables, and fruits).
- Limit amounts of solid fats such as butter and margarine and emphasize olive oil or other liquid oils.
- Emphasize regular physical activity.
- Use low-fat snacks such as pretzels, air-popped popcorn, low-fat crackers, and fruit.
- Eat desserts more like Italians do in Italy; rich desserts saved for special occasions with fruit served as a daily dessert.

AUDIOVISUAL AIDS AND SUGGESTED READING

EATING TO LOWER YOUR HIGH BLOOD CHO-LESTEROL. A booklet available from the Superintendent of Documents, U.S. Government Printing Office, Washington, D.C., 20402. NIH Publication No. 92-2920, Reprinted April 1992. Limited quantities free of charge.

THE LOWDOWN ON CHOLESTEROL. A 65-minute videotape on everything you need to know to choose a heart-healthy diet. Price: $79.95. Available from NASCO, 901 Janesville Ave., Fort Atkinson, Wisconsin 53538-0901 or call 1-800-558-9595 or fax 414-563-8296.

CARDIOVASCULAR DISEASE: NUTRITION FOR PREVENTION AND TREATMENT, 1990. By P.M. Kris-Etherton. A comprehensive manual for practitioners working with cardiovascular disease patients. Price: $42.00 ($35.70 for ADA members). Available from The American Dietetic Association, 216 W. Jackson Blvd., Chicago, IL 60606-6995 or call 312/899-0040.

DIABETES MELLITUS

SAMPLE TEST QUESTIONS

1. Which of the following is *not* a factor in the development of diabetes?
   a. obesity
   b. heredity
   c. insulin resistance
   d. excess muscle tissue *

2. When fat is used for energy, which of the following is excreted in the urine?
   a. amino acids
   b. ketones *
   c. albumin
   d. insulin

3. An elevation in the blood sugar level is called:
   a. hypoglycemia
   b. ketoacidosis
   c. hyperglycemia *
   d. hyperinsulinemia

4. The pills used to stimulate insulin secretion are called:
   a. ketones
   b. oral hypoglycemic agents *
   c. lente
   d. polyphagia

5. Diabetes acidosis is treated with:
   a. glucose
   b. candy
   c. juice
   d. insulin *

6. The management of diabetes includes:
   a. increased fiber
   b. increased complex carbohydrates
   c. decreased saturated fats
   d. all of the above *

7. The percentage of kcalories derived from protein in a diabetic diet should be about:
   a. 5 per cent
   b. 10–15 per cent *
   c. 20–30 per cent
   d. 40 per cent

8. The number of kcalories per kg body weight to maintain weight is generally:
   a. 10–20
   b. 20–30 *
   c. 30–40
   d. 40–50

9. Soluble fiber has been found to:
   a. help keep keep blood glucose levels normal
   b. lower triglyceride levels
   c. promote bowel regularity
   d. all of the above *

Match the definition in Column B with the appropriate term in Column A

A	**B**

_____ 10. diabetic retinopathy (d)

_____ 11. autonomic neuropathy (e)

_____ 12. postprandially (f)

_____ 13. peripheral neuropathy (c)

_____ 14. ketoacidosis (a)

_____ 15. polydipsia (b)

a. diabetic coma

b. increased thirst

c. nerve disease of the feet and legs

d. a disease of the small blood vessels found in the back of the eye

e. problems with the autonomic nervous system

f. after meals

---

16. The recommended allowance of carbohydrate in the diabetic diet is:
    a. 10–20 per cent
    b. 30–40 per cent
    c. 50–60 per cent *
    d. 70–80 per cent

17. The suggested intake of fat in the diabetic diet is:
    a. 10–20 per cent
    b. 20–30 per cent *
    c. 40–50 per cent
    d. over 50 per cent

18. Exercise can lower blood glucose levels as long as adequate amounts of _____ are available to the body.
    a. simple carbohydrates
    b. protein
    c. fat
    d. insulin *

19. Impaired glucose tolerance:
    a. is related to cardiovascular disease
    b. was formerly known as borderline diabetes
    c. often co-exists with hypertriglyceridemia
    d. all of the above *

20. Insulin is composed of:
    a. protein *
    b. enzymes
    c. sugar
    d. triglycerides

21. Insulin is produced in the:
    a. liver
    b. pancreas *
    c. stomach
    d. intestine

22. Stress can lead to hyperglycemia by causing the liver to release:
    a. insulin
    b. ketones
    c. fructose
    d. glucose from glycogen stores *

23. The warning signs of diabetes include:
    a. unexplained weight loss
    b. increased appetite
    c. unusual thirst
    d. all of the above *

24. If alcohol is consumed with diabetes it should:
    a. be in moderate amounts only
    b. not include sweet liquers
    c. be consumed along with complex carbohydrate foods
    d. all of the above *

25. Factors that raise blood sugar levels include:
    a. stress such as illness or surgery
    b. both simple and complex carbohydrates
    c. pregnancy
    d. all of the above *

INSTRUCTIONAL POINTS ON "A FAMILY'S PERSPECTIVE ON NUTRITION"

- Ask students if they would give up a piece of birthday cake if they had diabetes.
- Do any of the students have family or friends with diabetes? What kinds of decisions do they have to make?
- Ask students how they feel regarding the class activity on checking their own blood sugars (see Study Questions and Activities at the end of the text chapter). Are they apprehensive? How might a patient feel if he or she was asked to check daily blood sugar levels?

ANSWERS TO TEXTBOOK STUDY QUESTIONS AND ACTIVITIES

1. Advice for Mr. Bernardo regarding eating foods such as pizza, lasagna, or dried fruit:
   Pizza
   - Avoid extra or double cheese
   - Avoid high fat meat toppings (sausage and pepperoni)
   - Order pizza without mozzarella or with low-fat mozzarella if possible
   - Order with vegetable toppings (mushrooms, green pepper, onion, and so on)
   - Make pizza at home using oatbran in place of some flour for increased soluble fiber
   - Limit to two large slices and include a salad to fill up on
   Lasagna
   - Use part-skim mozzarella and low-fat ricotta or low-fat cottage cheese
   - Have meatless lasagna or use lean hamburger or ground turkey
   - Add vegetables into the filling such as spinach or zucchini
   - Eat a portion only as big around as a sandwich
   Dried fruit
   - Limit to 1/4 cup to equal one fruit exchange (15 g carbohydrate)
   - Limit raisins to 1/8 cup (15 g carbohydrate)
   - Have dried fruit as part of a meal such as in place of dessert

2. To calculate known carbohydrate, protein, and fat content of a given food into exchanges, determine the most appropriate food categories and mathematically estimate as close as possible. For example, one serving of fish sticks contains 10 g protein, 20 g carbohydrate, and 14 g fat. This approximately equals one high-fat meat exchange, one bread exchange, and one fat exchange (10 g protein, 15 g carbohydrate, and 13 g fat).

3. No correct answer; have students discuss their reactions.

4. No correct answer; have students discuss their reactions. Have students list some of their favorite high fat/ high sugar foods and snacks and ask for their reaction if they were told not to eat these foods.

5. Some possible reasons for elevated blood glucose levels:
   - Changes in diet with increased carbohydrate intake (especially simple carbohydrates)
   - Increased stress levels
   - Infection or illness
   - Decreased exercise level

6. Elevated lipids often are associated with diabetes, especially if it is uncontrolled. This is associated with heart disease. Small blood vessel disease is associated with kidney disease (and eye disease), which is in part related to elevated blood pressure.

7. To become a member of the American Diabetes Association, which includes a monthly journal, "Diabetes Forecast," write to American Diabetes Association, General Membership, P.O. Box 5014, Harlan, IA 51593-0514. The membership fee in 1994 was $24.00.

8. NPH insulin peaks in about 9 hours (although the human insulin tends to peak earlier), thus if a person takes NPH insulin at 7:00 A.M. the insulin will peak at the latest about 4:00 P.M. If the person begins to feel shaky at 3:00 P.M. he or she should check the blood glucose level and treat with 15 g readily absorbed carbohydrate if blood glucose is low (less than 60 mg/dl for a nonpregnant individual). The blood glucose should then be rechecked in 15 minutes (the 15:15 rule) and retreat with 15 to 30 g carbohydrate if it has not come up to normal limits. Once the blood glucose level is normal a balanced meal should follow such as a sandwich with a piece of fruit.

9. There is the equivalent of 3 teaspoons of milk sugar found in each cup of milk (4 g sugar equals 1 teaspoon sugar). Milk is less likely to raise blood glucose versus juice due to the increased digestion time of protein and fat.

10. A hyperglycemic patient with insulin-dependent diabetes mellitus (IDDM) who is determined to be a marathon athlete should:
   - Learn how to control hyperglycemia levels by consulting with a physician about insulin needs, a registered dietitian about diet needs, and learn how monitoring of blood glucose levels gives important data on which to make decisions regarding improved glucose control.
   - Undergo a complete physical examination to rule out other health problems such as autonomic neuropathy (in which the heart rate may not be able to speed up to compensate for increased oxygen needs with running) or proliferative retinopathy, which may lead to blindness with the jarring action of running.
   - Consult a registered dietitian (one who specializes in both sports nutrition and is a certified diabetes educator would be especially helpful) in regard to increased energy needs of exercise and the development of an optimal meal plan for the person.

To aid a patient with noninsulin-dependent diabetes mellitus (NIDDM) who refuses to take responsibility for diabetes management:
   - Assess reasons such as lack of knowledge about diabetes management or a belief that necessary changes are too difficult to make
   - Encourage involvement in a diabetes support group to learn from others
   - Evaluate hemoglobin A_{1c} levels to assess overall control

To aid a person with gestational diabetes who is losing weight as a result of attempts at following a physician prescribed 1,800 kcalorie ADA diet:
   - Explain that the purpose of the diet is to control weight gain and not to lose weight
   - Assess if the woman is monitoring her blood glucose levels and urine ketones (if not she should be in order to make appropriate nutritional recommendations—if there are no ketones in the urine the weight loss is not critical; if there are ketones and normal blood glucose levels the carbohydrate content of the diet needs to be increased; if there are ketones and hyperglycemia she needs to take insulin)
   - Encourage a slight increase of food aimed at increased vegetable oil (which will not contribute significantly to hyperglycemia)
   - Contact the person's physician about the weight loss and provide input on ketones and blood glucose values if available from the patient

AUDIOVISUAL AIDS AND SUGGESTED READING

LIVING WITH DIABETES: A WINNING FORMULA. Video produced for people with diabetes, their families, and for use by health professionals features interviews with diabetes experts plus celebrity Gloria Loring (whose son has diabetes), 35 minutes. Available from the Joslin Diabetes Center. Telephone orders (617) 732-2695; Fax (617) 732-2562. Price $32.95 plus $3.50 S/H.

GET SMART ABOUT DIABETES. 1994 Joslin Diabetes Center Catolog lists a variety of educational materials at affordable prices. Free by contacting the Joslin Diabetes Center at the telephone or fax number above or by writing to them at: One Joslin Place, Boston, MA 02215, U.S.A. Attn: Publications Department.

HEALTHY LIVING CATALOG, 1994 Edition. Publications and Products for People with Diabetes and Health-Care Professionals. American Diabetes Association. Lists a number of inexpensive educational materials. Call 1-800-232-3472 or write to ADbA at: 1970 Chain Bridge Road, McLean, VA 22109-0592.

STANDARDS OF MEDICAL CARE FOR PATIENTS WITH DIABETES MELLITUS. American Diabetes Association, Diabetes Care, 1991:14 (suppl 2):10-13.

NUTRITION GUIDE FOR PROFESSIONALS: DIABETES EDUCATION AND MEAL PLANNING. Alexandria, VA/Chicago: American Diabetes Association/American Dietetic Association, 1987.

THE SCOPE OF PRACTICE FOR DIABETES EDUCATORS AND THE STANDARDS OF PRACTICE FOR DIABETES EDUCATORS.

The Diabetes Educator, Jan/Feb 1992, Vol 18, No. 1.

A CORE CURRICULUM FOR DIABETES EDUCATION, 2nd edition. By V. Peragallo-Dittko, K. Godley, and J. Meyer. This is a fairly technical document that serves as the foundation of knowledge for diabetes educators. American Association of Diabetes Educators and the AADE Education and Research Foundation, Chicago, IL 1993.

RENAL DISEASE

SAMPLE TEST QUESTIONS

Match the definition in Column B with the term in Column A

A	**B**
___ 1. anuria (d)	a. a condition of protein found in urine
___ 2. oliguria (c)	b. excreted protein material
___ 3. albuminuria (a)	c. decreased urinary output
___ 4. creatinine (e)	d. lack of urinary excretion
___ 5. nitrogenous wastes (b)	e. a lab value used to assess kidney functioning

6. In the treatment for renal disease the following is recommended:
   a. 15 kcalories per kg body weight
   b. protein calculation is within the range of 0.5–1.5 g per kg body weight depending on the disorder *
   c. 200 mg of sodium
   d. free intake of foods high in potassium

7. The general guideline for restricting fluid with kidney failure is:
   a. 500 to 1,000 ml plus urinary output *
   b. 2,000 ml plus urinary output
   c. 100 ml plus urinary output
   d. 2,500 ml plus urinary output

8. Renal disease often liberalizes intake of:
   a. sugar and unsaturated fats *
   b. protein
   c. kcalories
   d. potassium and sodium

9. Calcium oxalate kidney stone formation is related to:
   a. oxalate intake binding with calcium *
   b. a low protein intake
   c. a high calcium intake
   d. none of the above

10. Carnitine is produced in the:
    a. heart
    b. gallbladder
    c. bladder
    d. kidneys *

11. Hyperlipidemia associated with renal disease consisting of elevated triglyceride levels is treated with:
    a. a low-cholesterol diet
    b. a low-protein diet
    c. a low-sugar diet *
    d. none of the above

12. Osteodystrophy is caused by:
    a. low serum phosphorus levels
    b. high serum calcium levels
    c. a combination of high serum phosphorus and low serum calcium levels with altered parathyroid function *
    d. low urinary output

13. Dialysis is often begun when:
    a. creatinine levels exceed 15–20
    b. BUN is 28–50
    c. hemoglobin level is above 14 mg and BUN exceeds 20
    d. creatinine level exceeds 10–12 and the BUN is above 100 *

14. A vitamin and mineral supplement is:
    a. not necessary in persons with renal disease
    b. prudent for renal patients *
    c. recommended even without a physician consultation
    d. never recommended

15. The primary source of kilocalories for persons with renal disease and diabetes is:
    a. protein
    b. saturated fats
    c. complex carbohydrates and unsaturated fats *
    d. concentrated sweets

16. Anemia related to low erythropoietin production is best treated with:
    a. increased protein intake
    b. increased iron intake
    c. increased vitamin C intake
    d. none of the above *

17. Continuous ambulatory peritoneal dialysis:
    a. requires attachment to a dialysis machine
    b. entails filling the abdominal cavity with a fluid having a high glucose content *
    c. cannot be performed during sleep
    d. can never be used by persons with diabetes

18. Symptoms of uremia include:
    a. diarrhea
    b. nausea and vomiting *
    c. thirst
    d. increased hunger

19. Kidneys produce:
    a. bile
    b. amino acids
    c. renin *
    d. glucose

20. Supplementation during long-term hemodialysis with L-carnitine may:
    a. improve muscle function
    b. decrease hypotensive episodes
    c. improve protein catabolism
    d. all of the above *

21. The nurse can help the patient with chronic renal disease by:
    a. insisting on total dietary compliance
    b. insisting a vitamin and mineral supplement be taken daily
    c. providing positive reinforcement for dietary changes made by the patient *
    d. none of the above

22. Cranberry juice is recommended during renal failure because:
    a. it is high in acid
    b. it is low in protein, potassium, and phosphorus *
    c. it is high in vitamin C
    d. it is easily digested

23. Which of the following is sometimes liberalized due to hypotension of nephrotic syndrome:
    a. sodium *
    b. protein
    c. potassium
    d. magnesium

24. Health care professionals working with children with renal disease should:
    a. force the children to eat in order to promote growth
    b. not worry if a child with renal disease does not eat
    c. provide large portions so that the children can eat what they want
    d. make meal times pleasant and fun *

INSTRUCTIONAL POINTS ON "A FAMILY'S PERSPECTIVE ON NUTRITION"

- Ask if any students know of someone who has kidney stones or other kidney diseases.

- Have students discuss if they could have done what Rita Bernardo did—decline an invitation to a food treat. How do students handle such situations. Have any of the students eaten something they did not want or need just because it was offered? Discuss this situation in regard to other health concerns such as low fat for prevention of heart disease or weight control.

ANSWERS TO TEXTBOOK STUDY QUESTIONS AND ACTIVITIES

1. Foods that generally can be consumed freely include sugars and fats. The exception to this may be for a person with diabetes.

   Foods that should be consumed in moderate amounts include cranberry juice, lemonade, blueberries, grapes, lettuce, watermelon, and low-protein specialty products.

   Foods that should be consumed in restrictive amounts include protein foods (meat, eggs, milk, legumes), breads and cereals, and most fruits and vegetables (due to their potassium content)

2. Protein restriction lessens nitrogenous waste products. Electrolyte restriction helps prevent elevated blood levels and altered pH levels. Fluid restriction helps prevent fluid accumulation and edema.

3. Uremic symptoms develop when the kidneys cannot adequately remove nitrogenous waste materials and electrolytes with resultant build-up of urea in the blood and altered pH levels from excess electrolytes.

4. Students should be referred to the food composition table of their text appendix to determine the protein, phosphorus, sodium, and potassium content of their personal 24-hour food records.

5. Have students brainstorm some questions to ask at the renal dialysis unit that the class visits.

6. Fiona's snack, as described in the opening chapter case study, is appropriate for prevention of kidney stones. The mango chutney is low in oxalate content and the calcium in the cream cheese is not a concern. Assessment questions include determining how much fluid she consumes daily and to ask questions about the Digestive biscuits to determine their salt content, i.e., "Do the Digestive biscuits taste salty or can you see salt on them?" (They are in fact low in salt.)

7. Some possible explanations for Mr. Herman's behavior:
   - Denial of situation's severity
   - Anger and refusal to change his lifestyle
   - Lack of complete understanding of his condition
   - Coping mechanism, i.e., "one last binge"

Appropriate nurse response:

Sensitive communication to assess reasons for observed behavior with later follow-up as needed based on assessment. (To prevent a confrontation, this assessment might best be done at a later time. This decision requires a judgement based on Mr. Herman's nonverbal and verbal behavior.)

AUDIOVISUAL AIDS AND SUGGESTED READINGS

A HEALTHY FOOD GUIDE , DIABETES AND KIDNEY DISEASE, National Renal Diet, The American Dietetic Association. Similar to the Exchange List System for Diabetes. Available from the American Dietetic Association, 216 West Jackson Boulevard, Chicago, IL 60606-6995 or call 312/899-0040.

NATIONAL RENAL DIET: PROFESSIONAL GUIDE. Provides guidelines on use of the renal diet in patient care including addresses for manufacturers of special products. Price: $15.00 ($12.75 for ADA members). Available from the American Dietetic Association (see address/phone above).

GASTROINTESTINAL DISEASES AND DISORDERS

CHAPTER 11

SAMPLE TEST QUESTIONS

Match the definition in Column B with the appropriate term in Column A

A

_____ 1. achalasia (b)

_____ 2. cleft palate (e)

_____ 3. ascites (d)

_____ 4. cystic fibrosis (c)

_____ 5. gastritis (a)

B

a. inflammation of the stomach mucosa

b. the lower part of the esophagus fails to relax

c. insufficiency or abnormality of some essential hormone or enzyme

d. accumulation of fluid in the abdomen

e. an opening or hole in the roof of the mouth

---

6. Which of the following is *not* used to treat hiatal hernia?
   a. frequent small meals
   b. antacids
   c. bedtime snacks *
   d. surgery

7. Gastric secretions contain:
   a. fatty acids
   b. amino acids
   c. vitamin B_{12}
   d. hydrochloric acid *

8. Which of the following drugs is not used to treat peptic ulcer?
   a. antacids
   b. anticholinergic drugs
   c. aspirin *
   d. antibiotics

9. Which of these condiments is usually avoided by patients with ulcer disease?
   a. salt
   b. garlic powder
   c. cinnamon
   d. black pepper *

10. Caffeine-containing beverages are avoided with peptic ulcer disease because they:
    a. buffer acids
    b. dehydrate the body
    c. delay gastric secretions
    d. stimulate gastric secretions *

11. Steatorrhea is treated with:
    a. a low-fat diet and MCT oil *
    b. a high-fat diet with MCT oil
    c. a high-fat diet only
    d. a low-protein diet

12. Diverticulosis is treated with:
    a. a low-fiber diet
    b. a high-fiber diet *
    c. a low-protein diet
    d. a high-protein diet

13. In a gluten restricted diet, flours made from ____ are omitted.
    a. corn
    b. rice
    c. potato
    d. wheat *

14. In hepatic coma, ____ is (are) limited.
    a. carbohydrates
    b. fats
    c. protein *
    d. MCT

15. The nutritional problem that arises after a gastrectomy has been performed is:
    a. diabetes
    b. cachexia
    c. dumping syndrome *
    d. hyperinsulinemia

16. Dysphagia is generally a:
    a. stomach disorder
    b. neuromuscular problem *
    c. condition characterized by irregular contractions of the bowel
    d. condition in which there is excess hunger

17. Celiac sprue is:
    a. a condition affecting only adults
    b. a condition often found among persons of British heritage *
    c. a terminal illness
    d. treated with diet high in wheat, oats, rye, and barley

18. Symptoms of hepatitis include:
    a. weight gain
    b. constipation
    c. nausea and vomiting *
    d. hives

19. A disease of the pancreas is:
    a. hepatitis
    b. diabetes *
    c. ulcerative colitis
    d. lactose intolerance

20. In Crohn's disease:
    a. inflammation usually occurs in the terminal ileum *
    b. a low-protein diet is indicated
    c. a high-fiber diet is indicated
    d. a vitamin and mineral supplement is not necessary

21. Sickle cell disease is:
    a. a condition found mainly in children
    b. characterized by small red blood cells
    c. characterized by rigid, crescent-shaped erythrocytes *
    d. curable

22. An example of an organic stomach disorder is:
    a. indigestion
    b. peptic ulcer *
    c. hyperchlorhydria
    d. hypochlorhydria

23. The liver:
    a. concentrates and stores bile
    b. stores vitamins C and B_1
    c. stores glycogen and releases it as glucose *
    d. aids the digestion of fat

Match the definition in Column B with the appropriate term in Column A

A

____ 24. Peristalsis (e)

____ 25. videofluoroscopy (d)

____ 26. esophageal reflux (a)

____ 27. hiatus (b)

____ 28. mucosa (c)

B

a. the lower esophagus sphincter is incompetent

b. opening

c. lining

d. used to objectively diagnose dysphagia

e. a type of squeezing action of the digestive tract

INSTRUCTIONAL POINTS ON "A FAMILY'S PERSPECTIVE ON NUTRITION"

- Have class discuss Rita Bernardo's reaction to Dr. Shaw's age. How might his demeanor affect whether she follows his advice? How might the fact that Donna, the office nurse, being of Italian heritage, have positively influenced Mrs. Bernardo? How could Donna have used this same ethnic heritage to Mrs. Bernardo's benefit?

- Have class discuss how Mrs. Bernardo seems to rely on her son for his advice. In terms of fiber for diabetes versus diverticulitis how might his advice be contraindicated during the inflammation stage? How might Donna assess this potential conflict of information? (She might inquire if anyone in the household was trying to eat more fiber for health reasons.)

ANSWERS TO TEXTBOOK STUDY QUESTIONS AND ACTIVITIES

1. A low-fiber diet would be recommended for Rita Bernardo during the inflammation stage of her diverticular disease (diverticulitis). Once the inflammation has subsided a high-fiber diet is recommended to help prevent the worsening of the condition by decreasing the pressure inside her intestinal tract (diverticulosis). Adequate fluid should also be promoted with a high-fiber diet.

2. Foods from Maria Bernardo's shopping list (refer to the opening case study of Chapter 3) that should be avoided by her mother-in-law during the diverticulitis stage include: capers, pignoli nuts, legumes, and frozen vegetables that have skin and seeds (examples: peas, corn, lima beans, green beans). After the inflammation has subsided (diverticulosis) legumes would be good for her to eat due to the high soluble fiber content.

3. Tissue in the liver is not able to function normally in cirrhosis and a 35–50 g protein diet helps build and repair the worn-out cells; it is the right amount to prevent both negative nitrogen balance and hepatic coma. If hepatic coma *does* develop, however, 0–20 g of protein reduces the toxic ammonia levels that affect the brain.

4. A low-fat diet is used to treat gallbladder disease because the gallbladder may not allow bile to be released properly to digest fats. (The liver produces bile but the gallbladder concentrates and stores bile for later release.) If gall stones are involved it may be very painful to the patient when bile is released for digestion of fats. A low-fat diet thus can help lesson the pain associated with cholelithiasis (gall stones).

5. A gluten restricted menu that meets the minimum number of servings of the Food Guide Pyramid:

Breakfast	Lunch
1/2 grapefruit	Sandwich made with
1 c. cream of rice	rice flour yeast
1 scrambled egg	bread, sliced
1 c. low-fat milk	roast beef, lettuce
fresh ground coffee	and and extra to-
1 tsp sugar	mato
	1/2 c. fruit cocktail
	1 c. low-fat milk
	fresh ground coffee

Supper

3 oz sliced turkey
1/2 c. mashed potato
2 corn muffins (gluten free)
1/2 c. peas and corn
2 tsp butter or gluten-free oleo
1/2 c. pure ice cream (no gluten stabilizers)
iced water

6. Five food labels that contain gluten are:
   - many commercial ice creams
   - wheat bread
   - saltine crackers
   - cookies
   - pudding mixes

7. A person with lactose intolerance can usually tolerate yogurt, lactose-reduced milk, and sometimes hard cheeses. Two to 3 cups of yogurt or lactose-reduced milk will provide adequate calcium for most persons. An ounce and a half of cheese is equivalent to 1 cup milk.

AUDIOVISUAL AIDS AND SUGGESTED READING

THE MILK SUGAR DILEMMA: LIVING WITH LACTOSE INTOLERANCE. By R.A. Martens and S. Martens. A practical handbook for individuals with lactose intolerance; includes a lactose-restricted diet sheet that can be copied for patient education and a comprehensive list of lactose-free food products and lactose-free recipes. Price: $13.95 + $1.50 S/H. Available from Sherlyn Hogenson, MS, RD, Medi-Ed Press, #5 Whites Place, Bloomington, IL 61701 or call 309-827-4620.

LACTOSE INTOLERANCE, 1991. By M.L. Dobler, R.D. A 21-page patient education booklet that defines lactose intolerance and its symptoms with food tips. Price: $5.50 ($4.65 ADA members). Available from The American Dietetic Association, 216 W. Jackson Blvd., Chicago, IL 60606-6995 or call 312/899-0040.

GLUTEN INTOLERANCE, 1991. By M.L. Dobler, R.D. A 25-page patient education booklet that defines gluten intolerance and its symptoms with guidelines for food choices. Price: $5.50 ($4.65 ADA members). Available from The American Dietetic Association, 216 W. Jackson Blvd., Chicago, IL 60606-6995 or call 312/899-0040.

CELIAC SPRUE ASSOCIATION/UNITED STATES OF AMERICA, Inc. Offers a number of free or inexpensive literature for patient use. Write them at: P.O. Box 31700, Omaha, NE 68131-0700 or call 402/558-0600.

A BASIC PRIMER ON CELIAC DISEASE. A videocassette from Celiac Sprue Association. Price $16.00. Order using above address/phone number.

CHAPTER 12

NUTRITION AND CANCER

SAMPLE TEST QUESTIONS

1. The study of tumors is called:
   a. pharmacology
   b. flexicology
   c. oncology *
   d. none of the above

2. Cancer cachexia is a condition related to:
   a. good nutritional status
   b. vitamin C deficiency
   c. malnutrition and emaciation *
   d. all of the above

3. Cachexia may develop due to:
   a. altered sense of taste
   b. an early feeling of fullness
   c. nausea and vomiting
   d. all of the above *

4. A person who has throat cancer and is treated with radiation therapy is at high risk of:
   a. severe dental caries *
   b. lung disease
   c. heart disease
   d. blindness

5. Steroids used in chemotherapy may require:
   a. a decreased intake of sodium and simple carbohydrates *
   b. an increased intake of sodium and simple carbohydrates
   c. only a sodium restriction
   d. only a carbohydrate restriction

6. Nutritional goals during cancer treatment are:
   a. prevention of weight loss
   b. controlling electrolyte loss due to nausea and vomiting
   c. providing at least the RDA for all nutrients
   d. all of the above *

7. Cancer prevention can be promoted nutritionally by:
   a. reducing saturated fat intake
   b. having only moderate alcohol intake
   c. increasing fiber through whole grains, vegetables, and fruits
   d. all of the above *

8. A malignant tumor:
   a. takes away the food and blood supply from normal cells *
   b. will not spread to other parts of the body
   c. is only caused from excess sun exposure
   d. can be cured with a macrobiotic diet

9. A person with cancer may need as many kcalories and protein as _____ to prevent weight loss.
   a. 1,000 kcalories and 45 g protein
   b. 1,500 kcalories and 60 g protein
   c. 3,000 to 4,000 kcalories and 100 to 200 g protein *
   d. 5,000 to 6,000 kcalories and 200 to 300 g protein

10. Frequently reported symptoms affecting eating with cancer are:
    a. alterations in taste and smell
    b. a high threshold for tasting sweets
    c. both a and b *
    d. neither a nor b

11. A person with cancer who is overweight should be instructed on a weight loss plan:
    a. true
    b. false *

12. A fiber intake of 20 to 30 g per day may help prevent both colon and breast cancer:
    a. true *
    b. false

13. Monounsaturated fats such as olive oil are *less* likely to promote cancer than polyunsaturated fats such as safflower oil:
    a. true *
    b. false

14. Malabsorption of nutrients may occur with radiation therapy to the abdominal region:
    a. true *
    b. false

15. The loss of muscle is not common during cancer:
    a. true
    b. false *

INSTRUCTIONAL POINTS ON "A FAMILY'S PERSPECTIVE ON NUTRITION"

- Ask students if they know where the Ukraine (a country that was part of the former Soviet Union) is and if they recall the Chernobyl explosion (a nuclear power plant explosion).
- Have students consider what it must have been like for Oksana, a new student from another country, to have an acute illness such as cancer. Discuss the biopyschosocial aspects of treating Oksana's cancer i.e., part of her weight loss may have been due to depression with all of these negative factors she had to contend with.

ANSWERS TO TEXTBOOK STUDY QUESTIONS AND ACTIVITIES

1. Patients with cancer experience anorexia for several reasons:
   - Altered sense of taste
   - Food aversions
   - A feeling of fullness
   - Nausea
   - Chemical substances produced by the tumor may affect the hypothalamus, which regulates hunger and satiety
   - Side effects of treatment often add to the patient's discomfort

2. The reasons listed in answer 1 also contribute to cancer cachexia; also, a lack of energy

3. Some of the nutritional problems imposed by cancer *radiation therapy* are irritation of the mouth, tongue, esophagus, and stomach; diarrhea, milk intolerance; nausea and vomiting, and malabsorption. Nutritional problems that develop after *surgery* include the inability to chew or swallow, dumping syndrome, diarrhea, malabsorption, and fluid and electrolyte imbalances. Nutritional problems associated with *chemotherapy* include others as well, such as taste, appetite, and weight changes. Dietary modifications such as small frequent meals, flavor enhancers, nutrient-dense liquids, and the avoidance of foods not tolerated may be recommended depending on the individual's needs.

4. It is important to individualize the diet of the cancer patient to guard against weight loss, which often leads to cancer cachexia and then poor response to therapy.

5. Now that Oksana is in remission from cancer, as described in the opening chapter case study, her nutritional goals include:
   - Regaining the lost weight from cancer treatment. Her Body Mass Index (see Appendix 16) should be in the range of 20–24 but up to 28 or 29 is acceptably high.
   - Eating balanced meals to increase her resistance to infection and illness. She particularly needs adequate protein to help

regain any muscle that was lost through weight loss. Vegetables and fruits are also very important as they provide vitamins A and C.

- Emphasizing low fat food choices with adequate fiber (as found in whole grains and vegetables and fruits), beta carotene (found in dark green leafy and deep orange vegetables and fruits), vitamin C (found in citrus fruits, strawberries, potatoes, green pepper, and dark green leafy vegetables), and cruciferous vegetables (broccoli, cauliflower, brussel sprouts, and cabbage), as these foods may help prevent the reoccurrence of cancer.

6. Case study with Mrs. Sweet:
Because Mrs. Sweet receives steroids, she may require a diet restricted in sodium and carbohydrate as a result of fluid retention and the potential for hyperglycemia. Her desire for sweets can be satisfied with the use of sugar substitutes. Appropriate sources of plant protein should be provided to substitute for the meat that she dislikes.

Nutritional goals for Mrs. Sweet:
- Maintain serum glucose within the normal range
- Provide adequate protein and vitamins/minerals
- Prevent weight loss
- Prevent edema

AUDIOVISUAL AIDS AND SUGGESTED READING

MAKING HEALTH COMMUNICATIONS WORK: A PLANNER'S GUIDE. By the U.S. Department of Health and Human Services and the National Cancer Institute, NIH publication #89-1493, 1992. Educators wanting to learn more about formative evaluation and qualitative methods in pretesting materials will find this useful. Call 800/4CANCER for up to three free copies.

EATING HINTS FOR CANCER PATIENTS IN TREATMENT. A 30-minute videotape that focuses on calorie and protein-dense food, how to cope with appetite depression, side effects of treatment, blenderized meals for swallowing problems, and cautions against nutrition quackery. Price: $79.95. Order from National Health Video, 12021 Wilshire Blvd., Suite 550, Los Angeles, CA 90025 or call 1-800-543-6803 or fax 310-476-0503.

CHAPTER 13

HIV AND AIDS

SAMPLE TEST QUESTIONS

Match the definition in Column B with the appropriate term in Column A

A

____ 1. AIDS (d)

____ 2. Karposi's sarcoma (c)

____ 3. Dementia (a)

____ 4. Thrush (b)

B

a. deranged mental functioning

b. an infection of the mouth

c. a skin disorder associated with AIDS

d. condition in which the body has lost its immune function

---

5. The general kcalorie demands for most AIDS patients is about ____ kcalories per kg body weight.
   a. 10
   b. 20
   c. 30–40
   d. 40–50 *

6. The term HIV stands for <u>Human Immuno-deficiency Virus</u>

7. The number of HIV-positive persons in the United States is estimated to be approximately:
   a. 1.5 million *
   b. 30 million
   c. 100,000
   d. 50,000

8. HIV is transmitted through:
   a. body fluids *
   b. handshaking
   c. drinking fountains
   d. all of the above

9. Diarrhea in the person with AIDS can result from:
   a. opportunistic infections of the GI tract
   b. medication side effects
   c. malabsorption
   d. all of the above *

10. Assessment of protein status can be determined through:
    a. lab values
    b. anthropometric measurements
    c. a diet history
    d. all of the above *

11. A high kcalorie intake is necessary if:
    a. there is fever and infection *
    b. there is constipation
    c. there is abdominal cramping
    d. there is dementia

12. The following is true of the person with AIDS:
    a. It is more difficult to regain lost body weight than to maintain body weight *
    b. A person with AIDS will only live about 4 weeks
    c. All family members of the AIDS patient are likely to become HIV positive
    d. Weight loss should be promoted for the overweight person with AIDS

13. Which of the following may prevent the person with AIDS from making good health care choices:
    a. weight loss
    b. thrush
    c. dementia *
    d. none of the above

14. The time of onset of AIDS after HIV infection is:
    a. always within 1 year
    b. variable depending on age and immune competence *
    c. immediate
    d. possibly never if the person eats well and prevents weight loss

15. The following persons are at high risk of infection by HIV:
    a. persons with multiple sexual partners *
    b. persons in a monogamous homosexual relationship
    c. persons using marijuana
    d. all persons living in urban areas

16. It may be determined that a person with HIV is consuming adequate kcalories if:
    a. the weight is stable or increasing *
    b. there is no anemia
    c. there is no dementia
    d. none of the above

17. Aside from a low-fat diet an increase in the following may help control diarrhea:
    a. oatmeal
    b. mashed potatoes
    c. banana flakes
    d. all of the above *

18. If a vitamin and mineral supplement is taken it should:
    a. contain 1,000 % of the RDAs
    b. be organic only
    c. supply 100%–200 % of the RDAs *
    d. be in conjunction with a macrobiotic diet

INSTRUCTIONAL POINTS ON "A FAMILY'S PERSPECTIVE ON NUTRITION"

- Ask students if they know anyone who is HIV positive or who died from AIDS.
- Discuss how heterosexual contracting of the HIV virus is increasing in incidence, while homosexual incidence is declining.
- Have students discuss why Denise is lucky to have a friend like Tony Bernardo. How might this friendship help her delay the onset of full-blown AIDS?

ANSWERS TO TEXTBOOK STUDY QUESTIONS AND ACTIVITIES

1. Nutritional management concerns between HIV and AIDS are:

HIV	AIDS
maintain stable weight; prevent weight loss	same
promote high nutrient density foods	same
add fats/sugars as needed for weight	same
	lactose-free diet for diarrhea
	soft diet for mouth sores or GI inflammation
	addition of soluble fiber such as applesauce and banana flakes to control diarrhea

The nutritional monitoring tool for Denise, from the opening chapter case study, is weight monitoring. If her weight is stable she is consuming adequate kcalories. Weight loss should send out the red flag for nutritional intervention.

2. A person with AIDS may need a high-kcalorie intake for the following reasons:
    • Elevated temperature due to infection
    • Diarrhea
    • Fat malabsorption

3   Diarrhea is treated in AIDS with:
    • Low-lactose diet (a common occurrence with GI inflammation)
    • MCT oil (for fat malabsorption)
    • Soluble fiber such as in applesauce, banana flakes, or in metamucil
    • Medication prescribed by the physician

4. For Mr. Smith to have an intake of 3,000 kcalories when he has mouth sores and no appetite he will probably require tube feeding. Ice cream, milkshakes, sherbet, custards, and cold liquid commercial supplements are most likely to be tolerated as the cold temperatures will be soothing to the mouth sores; but with no appetite it may not be feasible for Mr. Smith to consume this quantity. Monitoring his weight is the best way to determine if he is receiving adequate kcalories.

AUDIOVISUAL AIDS AND SUGGESTED READING

NUTRITION HANDBOOK FOR AIDS, SECOND EDITION. Provides professional information and ready-to-use information for clients. Price: $32.95 + $2.00 S/H. Order from: Carrot Top Nutrition Resources, Dept. CN, P.O. Box 460172, Aurora, CO 80046-0172 or call 303-690-3650.

NUTRITION HANDBOOK FOR AIDS UPDATE PACKET, 1992. Supplements the above Nutrition Handbook for AIDS with client handouts on dining out, beating fatigue, and questions about vitamins and minerals. Price: $8.95 + $1.50 S/H. Order from Carrot Top Nutrition (see above ordering information).

NUTRITIONAL SUPPORT IN PHYSIOLOGICAL STRESS

CHAPTER

14

SAMPLE TEST QUESTIONS

Match the appropriate definition in Column B with the term in Column A

A

____	1. hyperalimentation (d)
____	2. nutrition support (c)
____	3. phlebitis (b)
____	4. sepsis (e)
____	5. enteral nutrition (a)
____	6. aspiration (g)
____	7. physiological stress (f)
____	8. gastrostomy (h)

B

a. tube feeding or oral feeding

b. inflammation of a vein

c. the provision of macronutrients to promote healthy weight management and nutrition status

d. best used when the GI tract is not functioning or when there is severe vomiting

e. infection of the blood or other tissues

f. an insulin resistant state with increased amounts of stress-related hormones

g. fluid or liquid entering the lungs

h. a surgical placement or opening in the stomach for provision of direct tube feeding

---

9. Patients receiving tube feedings should be weighed:
    a. daily *
    b. weekly
    c. twice daily
    d. whenever there are signs of fluid retention

10. During the initial stages of nutrition support, serum glucose levels should be monitored:
    a. weekly
    b. monthly
    c. once daily
    d. at least two to three times daily *

11. Elemental diets are used in:
    a. short-bowel syndrome *
    b. hepatitis
    c. oral nutritional support
    d. cerebral palsy

12. The amount or rate of a tube feeding flow is determined by the person's need for:
    a. kcalories
    b. protein
    c. fluid
    d. all of the above *

13. For someone requiring 1,500 kcalories using a formula with 1 kcal per ml and a desired time interval of 12 hours per day, the rate of flow per hour would equate to:
    a. 100 cc per hour
    b. 125 cc per hour *
    c. 150 cc per hour
    d. 200 cc per hour

14. A common feature of commercial supplements for malabsorption is:
    a. MCT oil *
    b. bile salts
    c. high protein
    d. high carbohydrate

15. Manual delivery through a gastrostomy tube should take:
    a. 5 minutes
    b. 15 minutes *
    c. 1 hour
    d. 2 hours

16. Each kcalorie of supplement requires:
    a. approximately 1 cc of water *
    b. approximately 3 cc of water
    c. at least 5 cc of water
    d. no more than 1/2 cc of water

17. Commercially prepared formulas:
    a. are inexpensive
    b. provide a high risk of bacterial contamination
    c. allow the use of small tubes to administer the feedings *
    d. are inconvenient

18. Blood urea nitrogen values indicate:
    a. how the body is accepting an increased protein intake *
    b. the biological value of the protein found in the supplement
    c. a supplement that contains amino acids
    d. the electrolyte needs of the patient

19. The simplest form of peripheral parenteral nutrition support is:
    a. a liquid form of vitamins and minerals
    b. IV dextrose *
    c. used for more than 3 days
    d. all of the above

20. The most aggressive form of nutrition support is:
    a. hyperalimentation *
    b. peripheral parenteral nutrition
    c. between meal nourishments
    d. commercial liquid supplements

21. Recommended pregnancy glucose levels with nutrition support should never go above:
    a. 90 mg/dl
    b. 140 mg/dl *
    c. 180 mg/dl
    d. 200 mg/dl

22. The primary care physician and a registered dietitian should be alerted if a patient's weight drops to:
    a. 5%–10% of usual body weight *
    b. 15% of usual body weight
    c. 20% of usual body weight
    d. 25% of usual body weight

23. The physiological response to the stress of burns includes:
    a. edema
    b. high loss of nitrogen *
    c. damage to the gastrointestinal tract
    d. development of osteoporosis

24. In jejunostomy feeding, the tube is inserted through the:
    a. stomach
    b. mouth
    c. nose
    d. small intestine *

25. The following is an inappropriate time to begin total parenteral nutrition (hyperalimentation):
    a. when there is severe vomiting, concerns of aspiration, and significant weight loss
    b. when there is malabsorption
    c. for a terminally ill person *
    d. for patients with severe inflammatory bowel disease

26. If a person's blood glucose level is over 200 mg/dl the following should be done:
    a. decrease the rate of dextrose provided
    b. consider insulin administration, especially if glucose levels continue to rise
    c. continue monitoring of glucose levels at least two to three times daily
    d. all of the above *

27. To help prevent the refeeding syndrome the following should be done:
    a. monitor lab values such as phosphorus and glucose
    b. avoid excess intake of kcalories
    c. monitor heart rate, temperature, and respiration rate
    d. all of the above *

INSTRUCTIONAL POINTS ON "A FAMILY'S PERSPECTIVE ON NUTRITION"

- Ask students what they could do for Mrs. Bernardo if they were working with her. What kinds of conversational topics would be appropriate? Not appropriate?
- Discuss class reaction to the role of the dietitian in calculating nutrient needs based on lab values. Were they aware that dietitians are trained to do this? That a dietitian might advise a doctor on patient nutrient needs?
- How did the dietitian, Kathryn Wade, include other members of the health care team in her nutritional recommendations?

ANSWERS TO TEXTBOOK STUDY QUESTIONS AND ACTIVITIES

1. A high-protein diet is used to treat fractures, burns, and infections due to the tendency for negative nitrogen balance in stressful conditions such as these.

2. At 165 pounds Mrs. Bernardo weighs 74.8 kg. Using an equation of 1.5 g protein per kg of body weight this computes to 112 g protein (or about 110 g protein). This is probably not an excess amount of protein but lab values need to be monitored daily until verification is made. (Using the equation of 0.8 g protein per kg body weight is probably too low due to her depleted nutritional state.) Using the TPN regimen outlined in Appendix 11, this level of protein and kcalorie level of 2,200 is closest to D50W + 10 % Amino Acids delivered at 85 cc per hour (2,173 kcalories with 102 g protein). The extra 300 kcalories (to meet the estimated kcalorie need to promote a weekly weight gain of 1 pound as determined by the dietitian) is provided by added lipid emulsion (150 cc of 20% fat will provide 300 kcalories)

3. TPN was recommended over tube feeding for Mrs. Bernardo by the dietitian, Mrs. Wade, due to two factors: (1) severe hyperemesis with risk of aspiration and dislodging of a tube; and (2) severe weight loss of 10% of body weight

AUDIOVISUAL AIDS AND SUGGESTED READING

MASTERING THE TECHNIQUE OF TUBE FEEDING AT HOME, By Gastrostomy or Jejunostomy. Booklet available from Ross Laboratories, Columbus Ohio, 43216, December, 1991.

CLINTEC Professional Publications and Patient Instructional Materials available by calling Clintec at 1-800-422-ASK2, or writing them at Clintec Nutrition Company, Three Parkway North, Suite 500, P.O. Box 760, Deerfield, IL 60015-0760.

SUGGESTED GUIDELINES FOR NUTRITION AND METABOLIC MANAGEMENT OF ADULT PATIENTS RECEIVING NUTRITION SUPPORT, 2nd ed. By M.F. Winkler, MS, RD and L.K. Lysen, RD, RN, BSN. A pocket-sized guide provides an overview of enteral and parenteral nutrition followed by disease-specific guidelines that can be adapted to individual facilities. Price: $28.00 ($23.80 ADA members). Available from The American Dietetic Association, 216 W. Jackson Blvd., Chicago, IL 60606-6995 or call 312/899-0040.

PHYSIOLOGICAL AND PSYCHOLOGICAL FOOD ALLERGIES AND INTOLERANCES

CHAPTER

15

SAMPLE TEST QUESTIONS

Match the definition in Column B with the appropriate term in Column A

A

_____ 1. schizophrenia (b)

_____ 2. IGE antibody (e)

_____ 3. flight or fight response (d)

_____ 4. food intolerance (f)

_____ 5. food allergy (a)

_____ 6. anaphylactic shock (c)

B

a. a condition that develops when a person is hypersensitive to certain proteins in food

b. associated with behavioral eating problems

c. a life-threatening condition where the breathing passages are blocked

d. the hormonal response to stress that induces increased heart rate and blood pressure

e. produced in response to foreign substances

f. a condition that does not involve the immune system

---

7. The person with anorexia nervosa:
   a. is aware that the eating pattern is abnormal
   b. does not want to exercise
   c. loses control over eating
   d. has an underlying low self-esteem *

8. Foods generally allowed on an elimination diet include:
   a. meat, pasta, peas, and nuts
   b. rice, lamb, sweet potatoes, and carrots *
   c. cheese, corn, bananas, and sugar
   d. yogurt, egg yolks, white bread, and applesauce

9. Individuals who are sensitive to wheat may follow a diet restricted in:
   a. protein
   b. gluten *
   c. flour
   d. bran

10. Fat intolerance is often related to:
    a. cancer
    b. pancreatitis *
    c. peptic ulcer
    d. bulimia

11. Intolerance to hot, spicy food is often associated with:
    a. diabetes
    b. gallbladder disease *
    c. anorexia nervosa
    d. attention deficit hyperactivity disorder

12. Outpatient dietary treatment of bulimia:
    a. emphasizes regular meal times
    b. emphasizes food portions to satisfy hunger
    c. discourages food as a reward or for comfort
    d. all of the above *

13. All but one of the following is a symptom of hypersensitivity to food or foods:
    a. skin lesions
    b. gastrointestinal disturbances
    c. asthma
    d. fever *

14. A person with a milk allergy must avoid the following:
    a. cream soups
    b. casein
    c. lactalbumin
    d. all of the above *

15. A person with lactose intolerance is most likely to tolerate which of the following:
    a. ice cream
    b. soft cheese
    c. yogurt *
    d. chocolate milk

16. Anorexia nervosa does not occur in teenaged boys:
    a. true
    b. false *

17. Attention deficit hyperactivity disorder should best be treated with a sugar restriction:
    a. true
    b. false *

18. The diagnosis of food allergies is challenging to the medical community:
    a. true *
    b. false

19. The person with lactose intolerance will not be able to breathe if milk products are ingested:
    a. true
    b. false *

20. Adolescents with diabetes are at increased risk for eating disorders:
    a. true *
    b. false

INSTRUCTIONAL POINTS ON "A FAMILY'S PERSPECTIVE ON NUTRITION"

- Have class discuss how Rita Bernardo tends to rely on family and neighbor's advice regarding medical and nutrition concerns. How might a health care professional assess this tendency? (She might be asked who she talked with about her latest stomach ailment and what advice they gave her. This will help to assess Mrs. Bernardo's health beliefs.)
- Ask students how often they think people make changes in food habits based on advice given from family members or friends.
- Ask students to imagine they are a health care professional working with Tony Bernardo. How would they handle his request for advice on what his mother could and couldn't eat? (They should suggest he check with his mother's doctor as the diagnosis as described by Tony may be incorrect or incomplete.)

ANSWERS TO TEXTBOOK STUDY QUESTIONS AND ACTIVITIES

1. Symptoms of food allergy: skin lesions, hives, congestion, nausea, vomiting, headaches, and asthma.

2. The difference between food allergies and intolerances relates to the immune response. Allergies are immune related; intolerances are digestive related.

3. The symptoms of Rita Bernardo, in the opening chapter case study, are more likely to be lactose intolerance versus milk allergy due in part to the symptoms. The symptoms involved stomach pains with abdominal bloating and diarrhea. These symptoms were following the ingestion of a cream sauce and likely are related to the inability to digest the lactose. This is reinforced by her recent episode of diverticulitis with GI inflammation (see case study, Chapter 11). It is very possible in a few weeks that she may be able to again tolerate lactose especially if small amounts of milk are added to the diet to promote the reestablishment of lactose production.

4. The characteristics of anorexia nervosa versus bulimia are:

Anorexia Nervosa
severe underweight
insecure and introverted
fear of weight gain

Bulimia
normal weight or slightly overweight
self assured and extroverted
may or may not be afraid of weight gain

5. A day's menu for a person who is allergic to wheat and milk:

Breakfast
Rice cereal with soy milk
Fresh fruit
Fresh ground coffee

Lunch
Bean soup with rice crackers
Cornmeal muffins (gluten free)
Carrot sticks
Grapes
Iced herbal tea

Supper
4 ounces meat
1 c. rice with parsley
1 c. cooked vegetables
Dried fruit for dessert
1 c. soy milk to drink

AUDIOVISUAL AIDS AND SUGGESTED READING

BODY IMAGE THERAPY, A Program for Self-Directed Change by Thomas F. Cash, Ph.D. Complete audio program featuring four (60 minute) cassette tapes plus client workbook and clinician's manual, ISBN: 0-89862-965-0, Catalog #2965. Price: $35.00. Available from Guilford Publications, Inc., Dept. U, 72 Spring Street, New York, NY 10012 or call 1-800-365-7006.

FEEDING YOURSELF FORGIVENESS: A GUIDED EATING EXPERIENCE. By M.P. Gallant, MS, RD. A 45-minute audiotape for use with individuals or groups; helps clients eat more slowly thereby gaining more satisfaction from the eating experience; includes quiet music and relaxation techniques. Price: $10.95 (NY residents add 7 % tax) + $1.00 S/H. Order from Michelle P. Gallant, MS, RD, NUTRI-WISE, 2100 East Genesee Street, Syracuse, NY 13210 or call 315-428-0325

MATERNAL AND INFANT NUTRITION

SAMPLE TEST QUESTIONS

1. The growth of the fetus is affected by the:
   a. nutritional status of the mother
   b. nutritional intake of the mother during pregnancy
   c. neither a nor b
   d. both a and b *

2. Weight gain during pregnancy:
   a. should not exceed 10 pounds
   b. should be greatest during the first trimester
   c. should average about 24 pounds *
   d. has no bearing on the outcome of the pregnancy

3. A pregnant woman needs on average an additional ____ kilocalories per day versus the non-pregnant woman.
   a. 500
   b. 1000
   c. 750
   d. 300 *

4. Soy-based formulas are used when _____ :
   a. iron supplements are not necessary
   b. the infant is allergic to cow's milk formula *
   c. a formula low in phenylalanine is needed
   d. breast milk is unavailable

5. Cereal is given to the infant between the ages of 4 to 6 months in order to ____ :
   a. replenish the depleting stores of iron *
   b. satisfy the mother's need for sleep
   c. force the baby to eat more food
   d. none of the above

6. Breast milk:
   a. helps the nursing baby prevent infections *
   b. is harder to digest than cow's milk formula
   c. is more expensive than commercial formulas
   d. must be heated before giving to the infant

7. The ____ trimester of pregnancy is the critical period of embryonic development.
   a. first *
   b. second
   c. third
   d. all of the above

8. The recommended amount of weight gain for young infants is about:
   a. 1/2 pound per month
   b. 1 to 2 pounds per month *
   c. 3 to 4 pounds per month
   d. 3/4 pounds per month

9. The frequency of breast-feeding for the young infant is about every:
   a. 4 hours
   b. 1 hour
   c. 2 to 3 hours *
   d. 6 times per day

10. The let-down reflex is crucial for adequate weight gain in a breast-fed infant because hind milk is high in:
    a. fat *
    b. protein
    c. carbohydrate
    d. vitamins and minerals

Match the appropriate definition in Column B with the term in Column A

A

____   11. antidiuretic hormone (d)

____   12. fore milk (f)

____   13. immunoglobulin A (b)

____   14. hind milk (c)

____   15. pre-term milk (e)

____   16. colostrum (a)

B

a. substance that precedes breast milk

b. helps prevent infections and allergies

c. milk from the upper parts of the breast

d. regulates water loss through the kidneys

e. breast milk produced by a woman who is nursing a premature infant

f. milk from the front of the breast

---

17. Premenstrual syndrome is:
    a. caused by a poor diet
    b. caused by a deficiency of vitamins
    c. treated with diet therapy
    d. none of the above *

18. The pregnant teen who is at most risk nutritionally is:
    a. the teen who becomes pregnant close to the onset of menarche *
    b. the teen who is 15 years old
    c. the teen who is 17 years old
    d. the teen who is 19 years old

19. Maria Bernardo's baby Tony in the chapter case study:
    a. did not seem interested in being breast-fed *
    b. weighed less than 7 pounds at birth
    c. did not look healthy
    d. was bottle-fed because Maria was not able to breast-feed successfully

20. Gestational diabetes mellitus:
    a. is associated with birth defects
    b. increases the chance of having a large baby at birth if it is not controlled *
    c. may occur before the 12th week of pregnancy
    d. is diagnosed with a fasting blood glucose level under 60 mg/dl

21. The ____ is a product of conception that allows transfer of maternal nutrients to the fetus.
    a. amniotic fluid
    b. uterus
    c. placenta *
    d. enlarged breast size

22. Women whose weight is equal to 100% of the standard weight are advised to:
    a. eat twice as much as she did before becoming pregnant
    b. reach 120% of their standard weight at term *
    c. reach 150% of their standard weight at term
    d. gain 2 pounds per month on average

23. Overweight women should:
    a. gain no more than 15–25 pounds during pregnancy *
    b. lose weight during pregnancy
    c. gain less than 10 pounds during pregnancy
    d. gain at least 30 pounds during pregnancy

24. Excessive alcohol intake during pregnancy is associated with:
    a. fetal alcohol syndrome
    b. wide-set eyes
    c. mental retardation
    d. all of the above *

25. Maria Bernardo should be encouraged to do the following to control breast engorgement and soreness:
    a. use a rubber nipple shield
    b. try bottle-feeding
    c. use warm compresses just before nursing *
    d. use cold compresses just before nursing

INSTRUCTIONAL POINTS ON "A FAMILY'S PERSPECTIVE ON NUTRITION"

- Have class discuss how a nurse could easily talk Maria Bernardo into bottle-feeding (i.e., be a cause of breast-feeding failure).
- Discuss how emotions are very delicate after the stress of delivery. Ask students how they may overreact in a situation where they are overtired.

ANSWERS TO TEXTBOOK STUDY QUESTIONS AND ACTIVITIES

1. A well-nourished mother-to-be will benefit from good nutrition in these ways:
   - Have energy to cope with physical demands of pregnancy
   - Be less likely to experience nausea
   - Gain an appropriate amount of weight (not too much or too little)
   - Be less likely to develop pregnancy-induced hypertension (toxemia)
   - Maintain her health

2. Maria Bernardo's baby son's birth weight of 7 pounds, 10 ounces equals the 50th percentile, which is normal, and his length of 19 inches is at the 10th percentile. His length may be a reflection of genetics, assuming his parents are of shorter stature (if he stays at the 10th percentile for height until his 18th birthday his height will be 5'6½"—see older child's growth chart in the Appendix 13). His weight for height percentile is at the 75th percentile indicating good body stores. You can assure Mrs. Bernardo that her son looks healthy and with a good nutritional intake in infancy and childhood he may show an increased height potential.

3. The pregnant teenager should be sure to receive adequate kilocalories as well as sufficient amounts of all important nutrients both to promote good fetal growth as well as her own continued growth and to maintain her health. Because teenagers are at higher risk of having premature and low-birth-weight babies and other pregnancy complications, a good diet is critical.

4. Food needs are increased during pregnancy and lactation because of the energy demands of the products of conception such as the fetus, placenta, increased maternal blood supply, and milk supply after delivery. Milk or alternatives should be increased by 1 cup during pregnancy and 2 cups during lactation, meat or substitutes should be increased by 1 serving, and citrus fruit or other vitamin C foods should be increased by 1 serving during pregnancy and 2 servings during lactation.

   Maria's diet is already adequate to breast-feed successfully. She may want to emphasize milk for her bone health. She should avoid excess weight loss to ensure adequate energy to produce breast milk. Water intake should be encouraged but not be overly emphasized beyond her sense of thirst.

5. Alternatives to milk:
   - Lactose-reduced milk
   - Yogurt
   - Cheese
   - Pudding and ice cream
   - Soymilk and soy products (tofu)
   - Almonds
   - Sardines
   - Cream soup
   - Milkshakes and pasteurized eggnogs
   - Dark green leafy vegetables (except spinach)

6. The nurse working with Maria can support breast-feeding by:
   - Being empathetic
   - Encouraging Maria to try gentle hand massage to encourage milk expression in order to help avoid engorgement
   - With engorgement encourage a warm shower or leaning over a sink of warm water (with breasts in the water) to promote milk expression

- Encourage the use of cool compresses between nursings to control soreness (then use a warm compress just prior to nursing to promote milk flow)
- Encourage tapping the baby's feet to wake him up or gently shake him to wake him up in order to promote adequate nursing and lessening of Maria's engorgement.

IMMEDIATE CONCERNS FOR MARIA
- Breast engorgement inhibiting breast-feeding
  Solution: Warm compresses just before nursing to promote good milk flow, warm shower to promote milk flow when baby is not at the breast
- Sore and possibly cracked nipples
  Solution: Cool compresses between nursings to relieve soreness, nurse on the least sore side first, encourage short and frequent nursings so baby is not overly hungry (with vigorous suckling), expose breasts to air or sunlight to help healing of cracked nipples

LONG-TERM CONCERNS FOR MARIA
- Adequate milk production
  Solution: Avoid the use of rubber nipple shields and bottles
- Avoid confusion of baby between breast- and bottle-feeding (a different suckling action)
  Solution: Avoid all bottles, including water bottles, until breast-feeding is well established
- Likely concern over increased nursing frequency during growth spurts of infant
  Solution: Explain common growth spurt at age 3 weeks with increased nursing to every hour likely for a few days until milk supply increases "supply and demand"

7. Mrs. Bernardo can tell if breast-feeding is going well by the following indicators:
   - Nursing every 2–3 hours or 8–12 feedings in a 24-hour period
   - 6 or more wet diapers (assuming there are no water bottles)
   - Feeling the "let-down reflex" (a tingling feeling in the breast)

8. Growth spurts of baby Tony are likely to result in an increased demand for nursing. This often occurs at ages 3 weeks and 3 months but may happen at other times as well. This is Mother Nature's way of increasing the supply of breast milk through the increased demand (increased frequency). Frequent nursings at these times will increase the milk supply and baby Tony will again go for longer stretches of time in a few days.

9. Advantages of breast-feeding:
   - Increased immunologic resistance
   - Helps prevent allergies
   - Impossible to force feed
   - No special equipment needed
   - Requires baby to be held during feeding (good for the baby)
   - No need to mix formula or prepare bottles
   - No refrigeration required
   - Helps mother's body return to normal shape with uterine contractions and weight loss facilitated
   - Promotes a healthy baby

   Breast milk is suitable for the infant because it is easier to digest than other forms of milk and it contains all the nutrients needed for growth and helps prevent allergies and infections

10. Ways to encourage good food habits as baby Tony starts to eat solid foods are:
    - Wait until he is at least 4 months old
    - Do not force feed
    - Feed in a positive manner using a smile, verbal encouragement, and patience
    - Promote a leisurely meal such as by putting the feeding spoon down while he is chewing
    - Provide appropriate finger foods as he gets older (those that won't cause choking or those that are low in sodium and sugar)
    - Allow some food spillage when self-feeding begins, using an old shower curtain on the floor and small portions to reduce parental frustration

AUDIOVISUAL AIDS AND SUGGESTED READING

PRE-NATAL NUTRITION. A 14-minute videotape for $79.95. Available from National Health Video, 12021 Wilshire Blvd., Suite 550, Los Angeles, CA 90025 or call 1-800-543-6803 or fax 310-476-0503.

NO MORE MORNING SICKNESS, A Survival Guide for Pregnant Women. By M. Erick, 1993, 200 pg. Price: $13.50. Mail order to: Grinnen-Barrett Publishing Co. Box 779K, Brookline, MA 02146.

COMPREHENSIVE BIBLIOGRAPHY FOR HYPEREMESIS GRAVIDARUM AND/OR MORNING SICKNESS. By M. Erick, 1993. Over 450 references including international citations. Price: $16.00. Mail order to: Grinnen-Barrett Publishing Co. Box 779K, Brookline, MA 12146.

MORNING SICKNESS: ALL DAY AND ALL NIGHT. Videotape (28 minutes) featuring Miriam Erick with co-host reporter Liz Weiss, 1994. Price $79.00. Mail order to Grinnen-Barrett Publishing Co. Box 779K, Brookline, MA 12146.

BREASTFEEDING, SUPPLEMENTAL FEEDING, & WEANING. A 17-minute videotape for $79.95. Available from National Health Video, 12021 Wilshire Blvd., Suite 550, Los Angeles, CA 90025 or call 1-800-543-6803 or fax 310-476-0503.

WOMEN & NUTRITION. A 17-minute videotape with handout available for $79.95. Covers PMS, iron stores, dieting, osteoporosis, the pill, heart disease, and menopause. Available from National Health Video (see ordering information above).

GROWTH AND DEVELOPMENT

SAMPLE TEST QUESTIONS

Match the definition in Column B with the correct term in Column A

A

____ 1. adipose tissue (c)

____ 2. hematocrit (e)

____ 3. lean tissue (d)

____ 4. development (a)

____ 5. hemoglobin (f)

____ 6. growth (b)

B

a. refers to the increasing ability of the body parts to function

b. the increse in height and weight with age

c. body fat

d. muscle

e. the amount of packed red blood cells

f. the part of blood that carries oxygen

---

7. Snacks should be planned:
   a. from the six basic food groups
   b. only if the child has not liked the foods served at meals
   c. to add to the nutritional value of the diet *
   d. none of the above

8. Which of the following describes the eating behaviors of the preschool-aged child:
   a. strong food preferences and aversions
   b. a desire for simple foods
   c. food jags
   d. all of the above *

9. School-aged children need lunches that supply:
   a. one-third of the RDA for all nutrients *
   b. less than 300 mg of sodium
   c. 30 g of protein
   d. less than 5 g of fat

10. Nutrient requirements for children are based on:
    a. level of activity and chronological age
    b. individual growth rate
    c. both a and b *
    d. neither a nor b

11. Childhood obesity:
    a. is predictive of adult obesity
    b. requires that the child avoid all sweets
    c. tends to run in families *
    d. is not an important public health issue

12. Adolescent girls:
    a. have greater fatty tissue and less lean muscle tissue than do boys *
    b. have rapid growth between ages 15 and 17
    c. have less fatty tissue than do boys
    d. reach puberty after boys

13. To promote good eating by children the following should be done:
    a. encourage to eat alone to avoid distraction
    b. encourage to eat in front of the television for entertainment
    c. make mealtimes fun and enjoyable*
    d. none of the above

14. A child who is chronically undernourished is likely to:
    a. be sick more often than well-nourished children
    b. have anemia
    c. be shorter than well-nourished children
    d. all of the above *

15. In order to encourage eating of vegetables by children the following should be done:
    a. make children sit at the dinner table until vegetables are eaten
    b. do not give dessert until vegetables are eaten
    c. provide large portions so that some is eaten
    d. encourage to take one-taste of each vegetable served *

16. Terminology used with children needs to be:
    a. abstract
    b. concrete and non-scientific *
    c. as difficult as the child can say
    d. scientific

17. Barriers to good nutritional intake during adolescence include:
    a. peer pressure
    b. society's emphasis on slimness
    c. school sports and time conflict with dinner
    d. all of the above *

18. For increased absorption of the iron in cereal children should simultaneously eat foods high in:
    a. calcium
    b. vitamin C *
    c. vitamins A and D
    d. B vitamins

19. The following can lead to poor growth:
    a. anemia *
    b. puberty
    c. osteoporosis
    d. eating nutritious snacks before dinner

20. Breast-feeding should totally stop at what age:
    a. 1 year of age
    b. 2 years of age
    c. 3 years of age
    d. whenever the mother and child are ready *

21. If the child's growth follows the growth curve for both height and weight it can be assumed:
    a. the child is eating adequate amounts of protein
    b. the child is eating adequate amounts of kcalories
    c. the child is eating adequate amounts of vitamins and minerals
    d. all of the above *

22. The following children are at high risk for iron-deficiency:
    a. young children
    b. teen-aged girls who have started menstruating
    c. adolescents going through puberty and its associated rapid rate of growth
    d. all of the above *

23. Which lab values are used to help diagnose iron-deficiency anemia:
    a. hemoglobin and hematocrit *
    b. creatinine and albumin
    c. cholesterol and triglycerides
    d. serum potassium and phosphorus

24. Children, especially girls. just before puberty, tend to increase:
    a. their intake of calcium
    b. their muscle mass
    c. their level of body fatness *
    d. intake of fruit

Match the definition in Column B with the appropriate term in Column A

A	B
____ 25. food distribution system (d)	a. stop nursing or using the bottle
____ 26. subjective measures (f)	b. growth that occurs in length and density of bone
____ 27. bone growth (b)	c. overall deficit of food, especially kcalories
____ 28. food jags (e)	d. how food is allocated to the world's population
____ 29. wean (a)	e. eating only a few foods day after day or week after week
____ 30. marasmus (c)	f. descriptions such as "poor growth" versus "height at 10% for age"

INSTRUCTIONAL POINTS ON "A FAMILY'S PERSPECTIVE ON NUTRITION"

- Have students discuss their reactions to Maria wanting to breast-feed past 1 year.
- Could Rita Bernardo's perception of baby Tony's wanting to "nurse all the time" be biased? How does the stated frequency of Maria compare to this? How could a health care professional positively intervene in the family dynamics between grandmother, son, daughter-in-law, and grandson/son?
- Why was it helpful to Maria that her pediatrician warned about potential contrary advice from her mother-in-law regarding infant feeding recommendations?
- Can the students anticipate nutrition problems for the teenaged Bernardo children? What might they suggest to Maria before problems develop in regard to positive eating habits for teenagers.?

ANSWERS TO TEXTBOOK STUDY QUESTIONS AND ACTIVITIES

1. Growth: increase in size (height and weight) Development: increasing ability of body parts to function

2. Maria does not need to totally wean her baby until both she and the baby are comfortable with the idea. Most toddlers are self-weaning, meaning they need breast-feeding less frequently. Advice to Maria is for her to make her own decision. If weaning is desired, omitting one nursing at a time such as omitting the morning nursing is a positive approach. For example, baby Tony could be placed in his high-chair when he first wakes up so that he learns to eat cereal, fruit, or drink milk from a cup before he nurses. After he has eaten solid food he is less likely to want to nurse.

   Nanna Bernardo feels Maria is nursing too often, "all the time." This is a subjective description. Maria could more objectively describe the number of nursings per day.

3. A good breakfast is important from early childhood throughout life, because eating habits formed early can carry into adulthood. With nutrients missed from breakfast it becomes more difficult to consume enough later (such as calcium from milk).

4. If the Bernardos find it difficult to get their teenaged children, Anna and Joey, to eat an adequate breakfast they might try quick alternatives such as yogurt shakes or instant breakfast drinks added to a glass of milk. Allowing flexibility in choices will also help such as a piece of cold pizza or other leftovers from supper. Eating as a family is further helpful i.e., the whole family should plan to

sit down for at least 10 minutes at the breakfast table together.

To help 1-year-old Tony learn to eat new and different foods:

- Make it seem exciting to try new foods
- Offer small amounts of new food with well-liked familiar foods
- By example, demonstrate that new foods are tasty through facial and verbal expressions
- Encourage involvement in food preparation of the new food such as helping to put the food in the grocery cart at the store, preparing foods by "assisting" with stirring and pouring and so on.

5. Three lunches for school:

Tuna fish sandwich	Pasta and beans
Carrot sticks	Fresh orange
Dried fruit	Corn bread or polenta
Low-fat milk from school	Milk from school

Pasta with ricotta cheese
   and broccoli casserole
Italian bread
Milk from school

6. Expected effects in later life of inadequate quantity and quality of foods during the growth period:
- Poor growth (shorter stature and underdevelopment of muscles and organs)
- Poor development
- Anemia
- Poor dental health
- Excess body fat in proportion to muscle development

7. It is particularly important for an adolescent girl to have a good diet to prepare her body for reproductive needs, to replace iron lost through menstruation and rapid growth, and to promote good bone growth to help prevent osteoporosis later in life.

Some barriers to good nutrition that Anna Bernardo might face: pressure to be slim with diminished food intake, peer pressure and need for social acceptance regarding food choices, and rebellion against parental food preferences.

AUDIOVISUAL AIDS AND SUGGESTED READING

TEACHING CHILDREN GOOD NUTRITION. A 14-minute videotape for children grades 3 to 6. Price $59.95. Available from National Health Video, 12021 Wilshire Blvd., Suite 550, Los Angeles, CA 90025 or call 1-800-543-6803 or fax 310-476-0503.

CHUCKLEBERRY JOKES & SONGS AUDIOTAPE. Children will love to listen, laugh, and sing along with 18 simple and fun songs about good food. Price: $9.95 + $1.50 S/H; SPECIAL: Chuckleberry Tape + Joke & Songbook $19.95 + $3.00 S/H. Order from Laurie Manahan, Yummy Designs, P.O. Box 1851-CN, Walla Walla, WA 99362 or call 509-525-2072 or fax 509-529-8142.

GOOD FOOD PUPPETS & PUPPETRY BOOK. Make nutrition come alive with the puppet characters, "Mollie Milk" and "Frankie Fish" and others. Includes puppet lessons, activities, songs, and scripts. Set of seven puppets and Puppetry Book price: $59.98 + 15 % S/H. Order from Laurie Manahan, Yummy Designs (see above).

IF MY CHILD IS TOO FAT, WHAT I DO ABOUT IT? (booklet for parents) by J. Ikeda and CHILDREN AND WEIGHT: WHAT'S A PARENT TO DO? and FAMILY CHOICES FOR GOOD HEALTH (low-literacy booklets for parents). By J. Ikeda and R Mitchell. Price: $1.00 each. Available from ANR Publications, University of California, 6701 San Pablo Avenue, Oakland, CA 94608 or call: 415/642-2431.

CHILDREN AND WEIGHT: WHAT'S A PARENT TO DO? (12-minute videotape, includes sample parent books; also available in Spanish). Price: $35.00. Available from Visual Media, 1441 Research Park Drive, University of California, Davis, CA 95616.

SPECIAL FORMULAS. A 20-minute videotape reviewing special formulas for Cystic Fibrosis, Metabolic Disorders and other special health needs. Price: $75.00. Available from National Health Video, 12021 Wilshire Blvd., Suite 550, Los Angeles, CA 90025 or call 1-800-543-6803 or fax 310-476-0503.

TEEN NUTRITION. A 17-minute videotape that discusses the nutritional needs of teens and the dangers of chronic dieting. Price: $55.00. Available from: NASCO, 901 Janesville Ave., Fort Atkinson, Wisconsin 53538-0901 or call 1-800-558-9595 or fax 414/563-8296.

CHAPTER 18

NUTRITIONAL CARE OF THE DEVELOPMENTALLY DISABLED

SAMPLE TEST QUESTIONS

1. The term developmental disability refers to a severe, chronic disability that is manifested:
   a. before the person is 22 years of age *
   b. after the person is age 22
   c. between the ages of birth and 25 years of age
   d. at any age

2. Eating problems in the developmentally disabled population are caused by:
   a. anatomic defects
   b. mechanical obstruction of the oral and gastrointestinal tract
   c. behavioral problems
   d. all of the above *

3. Alterations in growth may be caused by:
   a. nutritional deficiency
   b. heredity
   c. chromosomal abnormalities
   d. all of the above *

4. Anticonvulsant medications increase the need for:
   a. vitamins A and C
   b. vitamin D
   c. calcium and folic acid
   d. vitamins A, C, folic acid, and calcium *

5. When chewing reflexes are lacking:
   a. hot foods stimulate them
   b. sweet and sour foods are effective *
   c. a pureed consistency of food is necessary
   d. only liquids are given

Match the terms in Column A with the appropriate description in Column B:

A

_____ 6. autism (d)

_____ 7. cerebral palsy (c)

_____ 8. neurological impairment (b)

_____ 9. epilepsy (a)

_____ 10. mental retardation (e)

B

a. a group of symptoms or conditions that overstimulate nerve cells of the brain, resulting in seizures

b. involves sensory, mentation and conscious functions

c. characterized by a persistent qualitative motor disorder caused by nonprogressive damage to the brain

d. characterized by extreme withdrawal and an obsessive desire to maintain the present status; temper tantrums and language disturbances are present

e. a general term for a wide range of conditions resulting from many different causes

72

Match the appropriate description in Column B with the term in Column A

A

___ 11. histidemia (a)

___ 12. maple syrup urine disease (b)

___ 13. ataxic (d)

___ 14. Down syndrome (f)

___ 15. Pradar-Willi syndrome (e)

___ 16. tongue thrust (c)

B

a. results in speech disorders and mental retardation

b. inability to utilize branched chain amino acids

c. a condition in which the teeth are not brought together to initiate swallowing

d. reduced muscle tone and growth retardation

e. small hands and feet

f. characterized by narrow eyes

---

17. Drugs used for controlling seizures include:
    a. anti convulsants, central nervous system stimulants, depressants, and laxatives *
    b. antacids and aspirin
    c. ferrous sulfate preparations
    d. diuretics

18. Galactosemia is characterized by:
    a. diarrhea, drowsiness, edema, liver failure, and mental retardation *
    b. a lack of an enzyme necessary to metabolize an amino acid
    c. a child with fair complexion and detached retinas
    d. spontaneous thrombosis

19. Homocystenuria is characterized by:
    a. a lack of transferase
    b. a musty or gamy odor
    c. eczema
    d. a lack of the enzyme necessary for sulfur amino acid metabolism *

20. The following conditions are associated with tongue thrust:
    a. obesity and hypertension
    b. Down syndrome and Prader-Willi syndrome *
    c. homocystenuria and galactosemia
    d. autism and epilepsy

21. The health professional who assesses oral motor function and recommends treatment is:
    a. the physical therapist
    b. the nurse
    c. the dietitian
    d. the speech therapist *

22. Persons with developmental disabilities often:
    a. have small hands and feet
    b. have small statures *
    c. are usually withdrawn and unfriendly
    d. are unable to live independently

Match the letter of the condition in Column B with the assistive device in Column A

A   **B**

____ 23. one handedness (c)   a. utensil holder

____ 24. limited range of wrist motion (d)   b. soft feeding spoon

____ 25. muscle weakness (a)   c. rocker knife

____ 26. bite reflex (b)   d. extension utensils

____ 27. incoordination (e)   e. covered cup or glass

Match the feeding technique in Column B with the feeding problem in Column A

A   **B**

____ 28. Rooting reflex (c)   a. placement of food should be alternated
                                        from one side of the mouth to the other

____ 29. bite reflex (d)
                                     b. use thickened pureed food

____ 30. chewing (a)
                                     c. avoid stimulation to the face between
                                        swallows or bites
____ 31. tongue thrust (b)

                                     d. wait for relaxation before removing spoon

---

32. Diet soda is not an appropriate reinforcer for:
    a. the overweight person
    b. the underweight person
    c. the person with phenylketonuria *
    d. the person with galactosemia

33. The following always increases mucus pro-
    duction and should not be given to persons
    who are congested:
    a. orange juice
    b. apple juice
    c. milk
    d. none of the above *

34. The following can be said about persons with
    Pradar-Willi syndrome:
    a. reduced kcalories are usually required to
       maintain a healthy weight
    b. persons with PWS are often obese
    c. food should not be used as a reward
    d. all of the above *

35. Food consistency for dysphagia should be:
    a. thin like water
    b. thick like pudding
    c. crunchy like raw carrots
    d. based upon an assessment of oral motor
       function *

36. Weighing a person with a Hoyt lift may lack
    accuracy:
    a. true *
    b. false

INSTRUCTIONAL POINTS ON "A FAMILY'S PERSPECTIVE ON NUTRITION"

- Ask students if they know any family or
  friends who have a developmental disability.
  Have they seen any documentaries or movies
  related to persons with developmental disabilities?

- Have students discuss why Maria might find her work so rewarding.
- Ask students if they are aware of how appalling institutional care of the developmentally disabled once was versus the more humane manner in which they are cared for now.

ANSWERS TO TEXTBOOK STUDY QUESTIONS AND ACTIVITIES

1. Down syndrome and Pradar-Willi syndrome are examples of specific diseases of the developmentally disabled population. The term *developmental disability* refers to a severe, chronic disability that meets the following criteria:
   - Attributable to a mental or physical impairment or a combination of mental and physical impairments.
   - Manifested before the person attains the age of 22.
   - Results in substantial functional limitations in three or more of the following areas of major life activity: self-care, receptive and expressive language, learning, mobility, self-direction, capacity for independent living, and economic self-sufficiency.
   - Reflects a need for a combination and sequence of special interdisciplinary or generic care, treatment, or other services that are life-long or of extended duration and that are individually planned and coordinated.

2. Nutritional problems are grouped as follows:
   - Eating problems
   - Alterations in growth
   - Drug/nutrient interactions
   - Weight control
   - Constipation
   - Dehydration
   - Dental problems

3. The growth retardation characteristics of Down syndrome:
   - Small flattened skull
   - Narrow nasal passage
   - Delayed tooth development
   - Narrow palate

4. The spastic type of cerebral palsy is likely to exhibit obesity, which may be due to limited movement. The athetoid type of cerebral palsy is likely to exhibit underweight, which may be the result of involuntary movements. Amy, from the opening chapter case study, probably has the athetoid form of cerebral palsy.

5. The students should be able to describe what it feels like to drink water in an awkward position.

6. Techniques used in feeding a person with tongue thrust:
   - Position client as described in the text material.
   - Do not let client push his or her head back.
   - Have patient exercise jaw control.
   - Use thickened, pureed food.
   - Place pressure on the tongue with the spoon.
   - Hold the pressure briefly to stop tongue from protruding.
   - Hold mouth closed until a swallow occurs.
   - If the person is a mouth breather, allow time for breathing between bites.

7. Appetite and behavior frequently are affected by the environment. Loud noises, bright lights, and sudden movements may cause the individual to become distracted from eating and become tense, thus affecting the mastering of mealtime skills.

8. When assessing the nutritional status of the developmentally disabled person, it often is necessary to use height rather than age as the index for determining the energy needs of a child when short stature is a characteristic of the condition. Bony deformities and severe contractures require that the person be weighed and measured differently from a normally developed person. Standard criteria for assessment are lacking for this population.

9. A person with developmental disability who also has hypertension needs to have the same nutritional goals as the general population, i.e., weight loss as needed and reduction of sodium intake. The dietary advice for such an individual needs to be very concrete. The person might be taught how to use the new food labels and only buy foods with less than the number 10 (10 % of sodium per serving) for example. The person might be able to be taught not to add salt at the table. Hunger cues might be able to be taught in order to

help the person avoid overeating, thereby promoting weight loss.

AUDIOVISUAL AIDS AND SUGGESTED READING

TOWARD INDEPENDENCE, Contemporary Products for People with Special Needs. 1994 Catalog. Includes a food shopping card set, recipe set, select-a-meal picture set, and other educational tools for the person with a developmental disability or for others who do not read. Available from the Attainment Company, P.O. Box 930160, Verona Wisconsin, 53593-0160 or call 1-800-327-4269.

PARENTS' VIEW OF LIVING WITH A CHILD WITH DISABILITIES. A 30-minute videotape with candid interviews with parents of children with disabilities regarding daily-life conflicts and dilemmas in dealing with health care professionals. Price: $95.00. Available from NASCO, 901 Janesville Ave., Fort Atkinson, Wisconsin 53538-0901 or call 1-800-558-9595 or fax 414/563-8296.

CHAPTER 19

ORAL AND DENTAL HEALTH

SAMPLE TEST QUESTIONS

Match the definition in Column B with the appropriate term in Column A

A	**B**
____ 1. cariogenic (d)	a. a build-up on dental surfaces
____ 2. dental caries (e)	b. brown mottling of the teeth
____ 3. dental plaque (a)	c. diminished or absent production of saliva
____ 4. fluorosis (b)	d. able to induce dental caries or cavities
____ 5. xerostomia (c)	e. cavities

6. Dental decay can be controlled by:
   a. limiting the frequency of carbohydrate snacks
   b. including a protein source at snack time
   c. the use of fluoride
   d. all of the above *

7. If tooth brushing immediately after eating is not possible then the individual should:
   a. chew gum after meals
   b. rinse the mouth with water *
   c. chew ice
   d. drink orange juice

8. Tooth decay is primarily caused by:
   a. loss of calcium from the tooth enamel *
   b. a lack of fluoride in drinking water
   c. not visiting the dentist for regular check-ups
   d. eating foods high in fat

9. Cheese as a part of a snack can help prevent dental decay because of its content of:
   a. calcium
   b. phosphorus
   c. fat
   d. all of the above *

10. Saliva production can be safely promoted by:
    a. taking an antihistamine
    b. eating crunchy vegetables
    c. chewing sugar free gum
    d. both b and c *

11. To help make sweet foods less cariogenic the following should be done:
    a. eat sweets between meals
    b. eat sweets before bedtime
    c. eat sweets with a pure carbohydrate meal
    d. eat sweets as part of balanced meals *

Match the definition in Column B with the appropriate term in Column A

A

____   12. purging (e)

____   13. dental enamel (c)

____   14. dental erosion (b)

____   15. periodontal disease (d)

____   16. decalcification (a)

B

a. removal of calcium from the tooth structure

b. caused by the action of acid on the teeth

c. the outer hard surface of the teeth

d. painless gum disease resulting in tooth loss in adulthood

e. induced vomiting

---

17. Joey Bernardo in the chapter case study probably had excessive dental erosion because of:
    a. his purging habit after meals *
    b. eating too many sweets
    c. not brushing his teeth
    d. using dental floss

18. During sleep:
    a. the production of saliva increases
    b. the production of saliva decreases *
    c. dental caries cannot develop
    d. the mouth is bacteria free

19. Breathing through the mouth may be a cause of tooth decay:
    a. true *
    b. false

20. Fluoride is helpful in preventing dental caries even in adulthood:
    a. true *
    b. false

21. Chewable vitamin C tablets are effective in promoting dental health:
    a. true
    b. false *

22. Saliva contains calcium:
    a. true *
    b. false

23. Hyperemesis can contribute to dental erosion:
    a. true *
    b. false

INSTRUCTIONAL POINTS ON "A FAMILY'S PERSPECTIVE ON NUTRITION"

• Can students determine what Joey's dentist figured out?
• In what way did the sport of wrestling adversely affect Joey's dental health?
• What should Joey's dentist do regarding his suspicions?

ANSWERS TO TEXTBOOK STUDY QUESTIONS AND ACTIVITIES

1. It is important to prevent baby bottle tooth decay due to:
   • Leaving adequate space for adult teeth
   • Enhancing a pleasant disposition of the baby
   • Avoiding a negative experience the first time going to a dentist

2. Joey Bernardo is at risk for dental erosion secondary to his purging behavior. Steps to be taken by:
   • Dental Hygienist—emphasize positive dental care to prevent further erosion/caries
   • Dentist—explain why purging leads to dental erosion and the impact of poor dental health
   • Parents—help Joey come to terms with his purging behavior and encourage a consultation with a registered dietitian to plan an appropriate weight control strategy. The parents should talk with the school coach

and other appropriate school personnel to help develop more positive weight control policies in wrestling and other school sports.

3. To help make snacking less harmful:
   - Brush and floss at least twice daily and ideally after each meal and snack
   - Regularly see a dentist for maintaining clean teeth (removing plaque)
   - Include small amounts of protein foods with carbohydrate foods such as cheese and crackers, cheese and fruit, peanut butter toast, or nuts and raisins

4. Fluoride tablets may be provided through the local health department via community health programs such as WIC, Headstart, or Well Child Clinics. Have students inquire about fluoride availability for persons who do not have fluoridated water.

AUDIOVISUAL AIDS AND SUGGESTED READING

SWEET TOOTH, 3rd ed., 1994. A computer software program designed for the secondary school level that illustrates hidden sources of sugar and tooth decay. Includes a diskette and user manual/teacher guide. Price: $39.95 (for Apple II series, and IBM PC series). Available from NASCO, 901 Janesville Ave., Fort Atkinson, Wisconsin, 53538-0901 or call 1-800-558-9595 or fax 414-563-8296.

MUNCHIES, 3rd ed., 1994. A computer software program designed for the secondary school level that helps students recognize smart snack choices by highlighting calorie density of foods. Includes a diskette and user manual/teacher guide. Price: $39.95 (for Apple II series, and IBM PC series). Available from NASCO, 901 Janesville Ave., Fort Atkinson, Wisconsin 53538-0901 or call 1-800-558-9595 or fax 414-563-8296.

MR. GROSS MOUTH™ MAKES 'EM GAG. A three-dimensional model of the teeth, tongue, and oral cavity graphically portrays effects of smokeless tobacco and shows clinical findings of gingivitis, oral carcinoma, dental caries, and gingival recession. Price: $89.00. Available from Health Edco, Education for Life 1993 catalog, P.O. Box 21207, Waco, TX 76702-1207 or call 1-800-299-3366, extension 295 or fax 817-751-0221.

DISEASES OF THE MOUTH. Slide or filmstrip shows tooth decay, gum disease, oral cancers, and general oral hygiene for grades 7 to adult. Price (slides): $69.00; (filmstrip): $59.00. Order from Health Edco (see above ordering information).

PHYSICAL FITNESS AND HEALTHY WEIGHT MANAGEMENT IN ACHIEVING WELLNESS

CHAPTER 20

SAMPLE TEST QUESTIONS

Match the definition in Column B with the appropriate term in Column A

A

____ 1. fad diet (c)

____ 2. anaerobic (b)

____ 3. Body Mass Index (a)

____ 4. carbohydrate loading (e)

____ 5. lipogenic (d)

B

a. a simple tool that more accurately determines appropriate body weight

b. without air

c. a diet that promises quick weight loss

d. promoting body fat

e. a method used to build up body stores of glycogen

---

6. For safe and permanent weight loss, a person should lose:
   a. 3 pounds per week
   b. no more than 1–2 pounds per week *
   c. 4 pounds per week
   d. 10 pounds per week

7. Vitamin and mineral supplementation should be ordered when energy intake is:
   a. less than 1,200 kcalories per day *
   b. less than 1,500 kcalories per day
   c. more than 1,500 kcalories per day
   d. all of the above

8. Which of the following requires the most energy to maintain itself:
   a. bone
   b. lean muscle *
   c. adipose tissue
   d. body water content

9. If weight loss is recommended to improve athletic performance:
   a. the weight loss should be quick
   b. a diuretic and laxative will be helpful
   c. fluids should be restricted
   d. weight loss should be gradual *

10. The adult energy requirement for maintaining weight with moderate activity is about ____ the basal energy requirement.
    a. 1 1/2 times *
    b. 2 times
    c. 2 1/2 times
    d. 3 times

11. During exercise most of the energy that is used comes from:
    a. protein
    b. carbohydrate *
    c. fat
    d. vitamins and minerals

12. Carbohydrate loading:
    a. is practiced mostly by short distance runners
    b. maximizes glycogen stores during an endurance competition *
    c. is achieved by consuming 100 g of carbohydrate per day
    d. decreases muscle glycogen stores

13. The suggested protein requirement for an athlete is:
    a. 0.8 g per kg body weight
    b. 1–1.5 g per kg body weight *
    c. met by taking protein supplements
    d. is best met by consuming 150 g of protein per day

14. A gain of 1 pound of body fat is the result of ingesting approximately:
    a. 500 kcalories above energy needs
    b. 1,000 kcalories above energy needs
    c. 3,500 kcalories above energy needs *
    d. 7,000 kcalories above energy needs

15. Permanent weight loss is best achieved through:
    a. reduction of dietary fat intake
    b. avoiding stress related eating
    c. exercise
    d. all of the above *

16. A common standard of obesity is defined as:
    a. greater than 5 per cent overweight
    b. greater than 10 per cent overweight
    c. greater than 15 per cent overweight
    d. greater than 20 per cent overweight *

Match the definition in Column B with the appropriate term in Column A

A

____ 17. hyperplasty (e)

____ 18. sports anemia (d)

____ 19. hyperinsulinemia (a)

____ 20. amenorrhea (f)

____ 21. hypertrophy (b)

____ 22. metabolism (c)

B

a. co-exists with obesity

b. enlargement of fat cells

c. the rate at which food kcalories are burned

d. related to an increase in plasma volume

e. increased number of fat cells

f. no menstrual period

23. Athletes require large amounts of protein for building muscles:
    a. true
    b. false *

24. Salt tablets are recommended for the athlete:
    a. true
    b. false *

25. Milk causes cotton mouth and should not be consumed before participating in a sports event:
    a. true
    b. false *

26. Obesity is known to cause hyperinsulinemia:
    a. true *
    b. false

27. Underweight is defined as being less than 10 per cent below recommended weight for height:
    a. true *
    b. false

28. A decrease of 500 kcalories per day from usual intake should result in a 1 pound weight loss in one week's time:
    a. true *
    b. false

29. Competitive athletes benefit from megavitamin therapy:
    a. true
    b. false *

INSTRUCTIONAL POINTS ON "A FAMILY'S PERSPECTIVE ON NUTRITION"

- Have class discuss how the manner in which a weight management class either promotes or discourages participation.
- What are the students' perceptions regarding an appropriate weight for Anna?
- How do students feel about losing weight without a "diet" sheet?
- How many of the class have tried a starvation diet or other diet in the past? Was there success or just a regain of any lost weight? How do students feel about weight loss in this society and culture that focuses on high-fat/high-sugar foods?

ANSWERS TO TEXTBOOK STUDY QUESTIONS AND ACTIVITIES

1. Joey's estimated kcalorie needs are 38 kcal per kg body weight while Anna's would only be 30 kcal per kg body weight. The factors having the greatest effect on energy needs include muscle mass (the main reason teenaged boys have a higher energy need than teenaged girls) and physical activity level.

2. Anna Bernardo's Body Mass Index is equal to 27 (draw a line from the height to her current weight using the nomogram in the text Appendix 16—the middle line is where you read the BMI). A weight goal of 100 pounds is too low for her as her BMI would then be 18, which is underweight. She should have a minimum of 1,200 kcalories per day to promote a sensible weight loss but 1,500 kcalories is probably more appropriate for a weekly weight loss goal of no more than 1 pound per week.

3. There are 160 kcalories in two slices of bread (30 g carbohydrate plus 6 g protein times 4 equals 144 kcalories plus 2 grams fat times 9 equals 18 kcalories for a total of 162 kcalories—160 rounded off).

4. The Bernardo family should use the Food Guide Pyramid as a meal guide. Separate meals do not need to be prepared. With emphasis on whole grains as the base of the diet, with plenty of vegetables, moderate intake of fruit, and decreased emphasis on meat and whole milk, and even less added fat and sugar, the whole family can benefit. The only exceptions are for the baby who needs whole milk until age 2 years and teenaged Joey who may need added oils to maintain his weight. By emphasizing olive oil for the fat source he will not be promoting heart disease or cancer.

5. A 1,200 kcalorie meal plan would contain:
   2 cups skim milk
   5 servings fresh or frozen vegetables and fresh, dried, or low-sugar canned fruits
   2 servings lean meat
   6 servings bread, pasta, and cereals

   A 3,000 kcalorie diet plan to promote weight gain should include six meals rather than three and contain at least:

4 servings fruits
4 servings vegetables
15 servings bread, pasta, and cereals
8 ounces meat or alternatives
4 cups milk

6. Role-play:

Mrs. Jones, RN, the school nurse, should describe the emphasis of a healthy weight loss plan and should use the minimum number of servings from the Food Guide Pyramid as the basis for food choices. Low-fat/low-sugar choices can be made. She can tell Anna Bernardo that this is her "diet plan."

The nurse can discourage Anna from skipping meals as a means to lose weight by stating that this can result in a decreased metabolism with an increased likelihood of overeating later due to hunger.

The nurse can advise Anna on a good weight loss goal by using the Body Mass Index. A BMI between 20–24 should be the lowest she should aim for (for Anna this would equate to no less than 110 pounds). A 20-pound weight loss that is permanent is a healthy goal for Anna. To attain this goal she should plan on taking at least 6 months to 1 year in order to best meet the goal of permanent weight loss (about 1/2 to 1 pound per week weight loss maximum).

AUDIOVISUAL AIDS AND SUGGESTED READING

EXERCISE AND WEIGHT MANAGEMENT and EXERCISE AND THE MANAGEMENT OF DIABETES. Videotapes for $79.95 each. Available from National Health Video, 12021 Wilshire Blvd., Suite 550, Los Angeles, CA 90025 or call 1-800-543-6803 or fax 310-476-0503.

HOW TO AVOID WEIGHT GAIN WHEN YOU STOP SMOKING. Videotape for $89.95 from National Health Video (see ordering information above).

THE HEALTHY WEIGHT: A PRACTICAL FOOD GUIDE, 1991. Price: $6.25 (($5.45 ADA members). Available from The American Dietetic Association, 216 W. Jackson Blvd., Chicago, IL 60606-6995 or call 312/899-0040.

CHAPTER 21

NUTRITION OF THE OLDER ADULT

SAMPLE TEST QUESTIONS

Match the definition in Column B with the term in Column A

A

_____ 1. gerontology (b)

_____ 2. aging (a)

_____ 3. geriatrics (d)

_____ 4. dementia (c)

B

a. process by which there is reduced capacity to replace worn-out cells

b. the study of the problems of aging in all its aspects

c. characterized by disorientation

d. concerned with the treatment and prevention of diseases affecting the elderly population

---

5. According to the Bureau of the Census, the number of people 100 years of age and older:
   a. is estimated to be approximately 200,000 by the year 2000
   b. is estimated to be approximately 100,000 by the year 2000 *
   c. will declinine by 1,000 each year to the year 2000
   d. will double between the years 2000 and 2100

6. As one ages:
   a. muscle mass increases
   b. bone density increases
   c. kcalorie requirements decrease *
   d. adipose tissue decreases

7. The protein requirement for a person over 51 years of age per kg body weight is:
   a. 5.0 g
   b. 0.8 to 1.0 g *
   c. 2.0 g
   d. 0.5 g

8. Women 51 years of age and older require:
   a. 0.8 mg iron per day
   b. 10 mg iron per day *
   c. 15 mg iron per day
   d. 18 mg iron per day

9. The elderly require a fluid intake of:
   a. 15 ml per kg body weight
   b. 20 ml per kg body weight
   c. 30 ml per kg body weight *
   d. 2 quarts per day

10. Fiber intake for the older adult should be:
    a. 10–15 g per day
    b. 20–30 g per day *
    c. 50 g per day
    d. 100 g per day

Match the characteristic in Column B with the condition in Column A

A

_____ 11. osteoarthritis (c)

_____ 12. gout (e)

_____ 13. osteoporosis (b)

_____ 14. rheumatoid arthritis (d)

_____ 15. Alzheimers (a)

B

a. characterized by increasing forgetfulness, disorientation, and behavioral food problems

b. develops gradually over a lifetime and may cause bone fractures

c. nutritionally managed by weight control

d. an inflammatory process currently best managed medically

e. characterized by pain in a single joint

Match the dietary considerations in Column B with the nutritional changes in Column A

A

_____ 16. less efficient digestion (c)

_____ 17. dental disease or lack of suitable dentures (d)

_____ 18. constipation (a)

_____ 19. decreased iron levels (b)

B

a. sufficient fiber and fluids

b. encourage intake of iron rich foods in combination with vitamin C foods

c. four to six smaller meals in a pleasant environment

d. foods may need to be chopped or pureed

---

20. Weights of elderly persons should be done:
    a. weekly in the home
    b. monthly in the hospital
    c. by using a calibrated balance beam scale *
    d. daily in the hospital

21. The Nutrition Screening Initiative:
    a. began in 1980 as a 5-year effort to promote nutrition screening and better care of older adults
    b. can be a way an elderly person assesses his or her own nutritional status *
    c. is a project of the American Medical Association
    d. Level II screen is designed for social service personnel for at risk persons

22. Meals on Wheels:
    a. is a federally sponsored program
    b. is a community-based program *
    c. must provide meals to all needy elderly persons
    d. must offer a congregate meal site

23. When serving a meal to an elderly person:
    a. address the person using the first name
    b. always cut the meat into bite-size pieces, butter the bread, and open containers
    c. provide adaptive equipment to help maintain independence *
    d. make sure the food is at room temperature to help enhance flavor

24. The amount of vitamin C an elderly person should ingest as foods is:
    a. 20 mg per day
    b. 60 mg per day *
    c. 1,000 mg per day
    d. 2,000 mg per day

25. The susceptibility to disease increases with age:
    a. true *
    b. false

26. Aging occurs at the same rate in all individuals:
    a. true
    b. false *

27. Arthritis can be cured with nutritional changes
    a. true
    b. false *

28. The physician should be the one to determine if a vitamin and mineral supplement should be taken by an elderly person:
    a. true *
    b. false

29. In pernicious anemia, vitamin B_{12} is given by injection:
    a. true *
    b. false

30. Steroid medication that may be used in the treatment of rheumatoid arthritis increases the need for:
    a. vitamins C and D
    b. pyridoxine and folate
    c. calcium and phosphorus
    d. all of the above *

INSTRUCTIONAL POINTS ON "A FAMILY'S PERSPECTIVE ON NUTRITION"

- How do students feel about Mabel Campbell having to sell her farm in order to be cared for in a nursing home with Medicaid funds? Are students aware that a large portion of the Medicaid funding goes to long-term care?
- What kind of visions might the students have regarding affordable long-term care? What thoughts do they have for themselves when they reach the age or health status of dependency on others?

ANSWERS TO TEXTBOOK STUDY QUESTIONS AND ACTIVITIES

1. It is necessary for the health professional to understand the physiologic changes that occur with aging in order to deal with the many nutritional problems the elderly experience. Perceptual problems, immobility, constipation, dental problems, digestive difficulties, and decreased tolerance to fat and lactose are a few of the nutritional problems that could be managed better if the physiologic changes are understood.

2. The elderly are vulnerable to nutritional deficiencies because of increased susceptibility to chronic diseases and because of decreased functioning of body organs, which adversely affects the absorption, transportation, metabolism, and excretion of essential nutrients.

3. Nutrition programs for the elderly have helped to improve the nutritional status of this population by providing meals that contain one-third of the RDA of nutrients. The programs also provide transportation to senior centers, health services, and recreational activities, as well as nutrition education.

4. After observing the meal service at a local nursing home, the students should be able to describe the residents' responses to the meals served and describe how meals were modified to meet specific needs of individuals. The students could discuss the role of staff in creating a pleasant dining atmosphere.

5. This activity helps point out the importance of patience and understanding when feeding a visually impaired elderly person. The blindfolded student will realize the importance of having the food described before tasting as well as the need to be kept from being messy.

6. Appropriate nutritional advice for an overweight widower with hypertension and elevated cholesterol with the need to rely on convenience foods should be centered around the guidelines of the Food Guide Pyramid. The guidelines are as follows:
   - Emphasize whole grains as the base of the diet (such as bread and cereal) with no more than 150 mg sodium per serving

- Focus on frozen vegetables (if the widower has a microwave oven preparation is minimal); all fruits are fine but should be packed in light syrup or in its own juice for less sugar (kcalories)
- Lean fresh meat such as skinned, boneless chicken breasts, ground turkey, or lean hamburger requires little preparation and is appropriate in moderate amounts (no more than 6 ounces per day—the size of two decks of cards total for the day)
- Use 1% or skim milk or non-fat yogurt, low-fat cheese should be kept to a maximum of 2 ounces per day to avoid excess salt intake
- Use minimal amounts of added fat with focus on liquid oils to promote decreased cholesterol levels
- For prepared convenience foods the widower can use the following guidelines in reading food labels:

  < 20 g fat per meal serving; < 2 g fat per snack serving

  < 800 mg sodium per meal serving; < 150 mg sodium per snack serving

7. Possible nutritional concerns of Mrs. Campbell from the opening chapter case study include concerns of food pouching due to the Alzheimer's disease, weight loss from not eating on her own accord, increased risk of dental decay and infection from pouching and due to probable poor dental hygiene, and increased risk of infection such as pneumonia with any significant weight loss.

AUDIOVISUAL AIDS AND SUGGESTED READING

NUTRITION FOR THE OVER-50 GANG. A 15-minute videotape available from National Health Video, 12021 Wilshire Blvd. Suite 550, Los Angeles, CA 90025. Price: $79.95.

NUTRITION CARE IN NURSING FACILITIES. By C.L. Gerwick, 1992. Price: $28.00 ($24.00 ADA members). Covers nutrition assessment and screening, risk factors associated with poor nutritional status in older adults, team approaches to care planning, and issues related to quality of life and feeding the terminally ill. Available from the American Dietetic Association, 216 W. Jackson Blvd., Chicago, IL 60606-6995 or call 312/899-0040.

NATIONAL AND INTERNATIONAL NUTRITION PROGRAMS AND CONCERNS

SAMPLE TEST QUESTIONS

Match the definition in Column B with the appropriate term in Column A

A

_____ 1. ambulatory care (c)

_____ 2. palliative care (a)

_____ 3. hospices (d)

_____ 4. holistic (b)

B

a. noncurative

b. takes into account all aspects of a person's health

c. health care in a noninstitutional setting

d. support services for terminally ill persons and their families

---

5. In less developed countries, nutrition problems are greatest among:
   a. women and children *
   b. those over 60 years of age
   c. teenagers
   d. working women

6. The organization that had been helpful to Maria Bernardo in maintaining breast-feeding in the opening case-study was:
   a. the EFNEP program
   b. the La Leche League *
   c. the WIC program
   d. the Food Stamp program

7. Forty per cent of the persons living in poverty are:
   a. unemployed men
   b. unemployed women
   c. elderly persons
   d. children *

8. Project Head Start is aimed at children ages:
   a. 1–3
   b. 3–5 *
   c. 5–7
   d. 7–10

9. The following persons may receive WIC benefits for children up to age 5 years:
   a. mothers of the children
   b. fathers of the children
   c. foster parents
   d. all of the above *

Match the purpose in Column B with the appropriate organization in Column A

A	B

A

____ 10. World Health Organization (WHO) (c)

____ 11. United Nations Food and Agriculture Organization (FAO) (a)

____ 12. UNICEF (b)

____ 13. World Bank (d)

B

a. studies aspects of world food problems

b. directs the distribution of milk to children worldwide

c. focuses on worldwide nutrition and health problems

d. sponsors international projects through agricultural and nutritional divisions

---

Match the definition in Column B with the appropriate term in Column A

A

____ 14. botulism (c)

____ 15. clostridium perfringens (b)

____ 16. salmonella (a)

____ 17. staphylococcus aureus (d)

B

a. bacteria widespread in nature that live in the intestinal tract of humans and animals

b. spore-forming bacteria that grow in the absence of oxygen

c. spore-forming organisms that produce toxin in the absence of oxygen

d. bacteria that are fairly resistant to heat

---

18. A food quack is a person who:
    a. makes claims contrary to accepted knowledge
    b. can claim to be a nutritionist
    c. may claim wholesome food is harmful in some way
    d. all of the above *

19. The WIC program:
    a. serves all women, infants, and children
    b. requires that participants have incomes less than 185 per cent of the poverty level *
    c. requires that participants have incomes less than 100 per cent of the poverty level
    d. does not prescribe supplemental foods to help the growth of children

20. Foods should not be kept at room temperature, including preparation and serving time, more than:
    a. 30 minutes
    b. 1 hour
    c. 2 hours *
    d. 4 hours

21. Why should health care providers be involved in legislative advocacy?
    a. inequitable food distribution system
    b. health care becoming business oriented
    c. increasing levels of poverty and risk of hunger and malnutrition
    d. all of the above *

22. The USDA conducts a food consumption survey approximately:
    a. every 2 years
    b. every 5 years
    c. every 10 years *
    d. as needed

23. The number of persons estimated to be eligible for food stamps is:
    a. 10 million
    b. 20 to 25 million
    c. 35 to 40 million *
    d. 50 to 60 million

24. The following can be said about the food shopping habits of persons receiving food stamps:
    a. the food shopping habits are generally as good or better than persons not needing food stamps
    b. low-income households generally have a higher nutrient return per dollar
    c. both a and b *
    d. neither a nor b

25. Tony Bernardo, in the opening case study, was able to bring his cholesterol and triglycerides level below 200:
    a. true *
    b. false

26. The Nutrition Program for the Elderly provides congregate meal sites and home-delivered meals to homebound elderly persons:
    a. true *
    b. false

27. The Expanded Food and Nutrition Education Program (EFNEP) offers home-based nutrition education for low-income families:
    a. true *
    b. false

28. The high-risk temperature zone for causing food poisoning is:
    a. between 0 and 32 degrees Fahrenheit
    b. between 32 and 40 degrees Fahrenheit
    c. between 40 and 140 degrees Fahrenheit *
    d. between 140 and 180 degrees Fahrenheit

Match the use in Column B with the appropriate additive in Column A

A

_____ 29. stabilizers and thickeners (f)

_____ 30. niacin (d)

_____ 31. spices (a)

_____ 32. leavening agents (b)

_____ 33. anti-oxidants (c)

_____ 34. humectants (e)

B

a. gives a variety of flavors to cakes and sausages

b. to provide desired texture

c. keep fats from turning rancid and certain fresh fruits from darkening during processing

d. to improve nutritional value of breads and cereals

e. distribute tiny particles of one liquid in another to improve texture and consistency

f. give smooth, uniform texture, flavor, and desired consistency

---

INSTRUCTIONAL POINTS ON "A FAMILY'S PERSPECTIVE ON NUTRITION"

- How do the students feel about the nutrition and health programs used by the Bernardo family?
- How does the class feel about the Food Stamp Program?
- Have students reflect on Maria's year from her hyperemesis to a difficult time initiating breast-feeding to her current day and outlook for the future.

ANSWERS TO TEXTBOOK STUDY QUESTIONS AND ACTIVITIES

1. The community programs that were helpful to the Bernardo's as described in the opening chapter case study were:
   - The La Leche League
   - The American Cancer Society
   - The Employee Assistance Program
   - The Nutrition Program for the Elderly
   - Public Health Nursing
   - The WIC Supplemental Nutrition Program
   - The Food Stamp Program

2. Legislation has affected public health relative to food and nutrition issues by setting federal standards on the public food supply to help ensure safe and wholesome food as well as to allow for funding of food and nutrition programs.

3. Existing food and nutrition programs include WIC, EFNEP, the Food Stamp Program, the Nutrition Program for the Elderly, and Project Headstart. Health programs include public health departments, well child clinics, health maintenance organizations, hospices, and other private programs.

4. An example of a food faddist is a person who claims to be a specialist in the field of food and nutrition and who exaggerates claims of the value of certain foods by emphasizing emotional appeal and stressing myths that other foods are both nutritionally inferior and the cause of disease and malnutrition.

5. Have students report on what they learned about nutrition activities of the local health department.

6. Students might briefly interview community nutritionists and dietitians to identify and describe organizations and nutrition programs available in the community.

7. The monthly income of the Bernardo family (prior to baby Tony's birth) to keep them above poverty level would have been about $1,400 but foodstamps are provided up to an income of 130% of the poverty level. (Rita Bernardo would have her social security income counted as family income since she eats the same foods as the rest of the family—the standard monthly social security income for a woman over the age of 65 is about $470 per month). Thus for a family of five (while Maria was pregnant) they would have had to have earned less than about $1,800 monthly to be eligible for foodstamps. Thus when Maria was not working Tony would have had to make less than an hourly wage of about $8.00 for a 40-hour week to be eligible for food stamps (which is not difficult to imagine since minimum wage is less than $5.00 per hour). To stay below 185 per cent of the poverty level this equates to a monthly income of less than $2,664 for a family of five.

8. Students can identify who their legislator is and his or her address and phone number by contacting their local league of women voters. The local public library may also be able to assist. Issues might be related to pesticide use or the need for insurance reimbursement of Medical Nutrition Therapy in order to promote dietitian services in patient care (currently very few insurance companies reimburse for nutrition services).

9. Have students describe their reactions to bacterial growth in the petri dish from the volunteer's swab of the inside of a refrigerator. Discuss the ramifications on food safety.

10. - Recommend draining liquid from canned vegetables and heat them in fresh water in order to decrease sodium content.
    - Suggest making homemade low-salt bread with donated flour.
    - Suggest soaking canned salty meat in water and drain before using.
    - Suggest using small amounts of canned salty meat in casseroles using low-salt pasta, potato, or rice.

- Explain canned fruit is low in salt, but for weight control, draining heavy syrup is recommended.

AUDIOVISUAL AIDS AND SUGGESTED READING

SAFE FOOD BACKGROUNDER. Reproducible consumer tips and question-and-answer documents for use in patient education. Available from Mary Young, Allied Health Education Coordinator, National Live Stock & Meat Board, by calling 312-670-9438.

FOOD NEWS FOR CONSUMERS. A publication by USDA's Food Safety and Inspection Service, available for $5.00 per year ($6.25 foreign) by ordering through: New Orders, Superintendent of Documents, P.O. Box 371954, Pittsburgh, PA 15250-7954 or fax 202- 512-2233.

FOOD SAFETY FOR PROFESSIONALS: A REFERENCE AND STUDY GUIDE. By M. McInnis and M.A. Keith, 1991. Price $17.00 ($14.25 ADA members). Available from The American Dietetic Association, 216 W. Jackson Blvd., Chicago, IL 60606-6995 or call 312-899-0040.

PESTICIDES IN FOOD: A GUIDE FOR PROFESSIONALS (Price: $6.95) and UNDERSTANDING PESTICIDES IN FOOD (for consumers; price: $10.95 for 10 brochures), 1991. Available from The American Dietetic Association (see above).

ADDITIONAL ADDRESSES FOR NUTRITION MATERIALS

All requests for information about audiovisual aids and other nutrition related materials should be accompanied by a stamped, self-addressed business envelope.

American Anorexia/Bulimia Association, Inc.
133 Cedar Lane
Teaneck, NJ 07666

American Association of Diabetes Educators
500 North Michigan Avenue, Suite 1400
Chicago, IL 60611

American Celiac Society
45 Gifford Avenue
Jersey City, NJ 07304

American Dry Milk Institute
130 North Franklin Street
Chicago, IL 60606

American Home Economics Association
1600 Twentieth Street, NW
Washington, DC 20006

American Institute for Cancer Research
803 West Broad Street
Falls Church, VA 22046

American Institute of Baking
400 East Ontario Street
Chicago, IL 60611

American Journal of Nursing
Educational Services Division
555 West 57th Street
New York, NY 10019

American Medical Association
Department of Foods and Nutrition
535 North Dearborn Street
Chicago, IL 60610

American Public Health Association
1790 Broadway
New York, NY 10019

Anorexia Nervosa and Associated Disorders
P.O. Box 7
Highland Park, IL 60035

Anorexia Nervosa and Related Eating Disorders, Inc.
P.O. Box 5002
Eugene, OR 94705

Best Foods
Consumer Service Department
International Plaza
Englewood Cliffs, NJ 07632

Breastfeeding Promotion Project
Seattle-King County
Department of Public Health
100 Prefontaine Avenue S.
Suite 500
Seattle, WA 98104

Child Food Care Program
Health and Environment Department
P.O. Box 968
Santa Fe, NM 87504-0968

Communications in Learning
2929 Main Street
Buffalo, NY 14214

Cornell University
Audio-Visual Resource Center
8 Research Park
Ithaca, NY 14850

Diabetes Center, Inc.
P.O. Box 739
Wayzata, MN 55391

The Food and Nutrition Information and Education Resources Center
National Agricultural Library Building
Room 304
Beltsville, MD 20705
(301) 344-3719

Health Communication Network
Division of Continuing Education
Medical University of South Carolina
Charleston, SC 29411

Health Learning Systems
1455 Broad Street
Bloomfield, NJ 07003

March of Dimes Foundation
White Plains, NY 10601

Media-Ed Press
P.O. Box 957
East Lansing, MI 48826-0957

Merck Sharp and Dohme
Health Information Services
P.O. Box 1486
West Point, PA 19454

Modern Talking Picture Service
5000 Park Street, North
St. Petersburg, FL 33709

NASCO West
1524 Princeton Avenue
Modesto, CA 95352
(209) 529-6957
1-800-558-9595

National Audio-Visual Center
Order Section
Washington, DC 20409

National Dairy Council
6300 North River Avenue
Rosemont, IL 60018

National Health Council
622 Third Avenue
New York, NY 10017

National Kidney Foundation of Massachusetts
344 Harvard Street
Brookline, MA 02146

National Livestock and Meat Board
36 Wabash Avenue
Chicago, IL 60603

National Restaurant Association
Educational Materials Center
1530 North Lake Shore Drive
Chicago, IL 60611

The Nutrition Foundation
99 Park Avenue
New York, NY 10016

Nutrition Today Society
101 Ridgely Avenue
P.O. Box 465
Annapolis, MD 21404

The Oryz Press
2214 North Central at Encanto
Phoenix, AZ 85004

Pennsylvania State University
Audio-Visual Services
State College, PA 16801

Photography Center Office of Governmental and Public Affairs
Department of Agriculture
Washington, DC 20250

Rice Council for Market Development
P.O. Box 22802
Houston, TX 77027

Ross Laboratories
Columbus, OH 43216

The Society of Nutrition Education
3140 Shattuck Avenue, Suite 1110
Berkeley, CA 94704

Sports Medicine Systems, Inc.
Nutrition Services
830 Boylston Street
Brookline, MA 02167

Stouffer Foods Corp.
5750 Harper Road
Solon, OH 44139-1880

Trainex Corporation
P.O. Box 116
Garden Grove, CA 92542
(714) 698-2561

U.S. Communicable Disease Center
U.S. Public Health Service
Audio-Visual Facility
Atlanta, GA 30301

U.S. Department of Agriculture
Superintendent of Documents
U.S. Government Printing Office
Washington, DC 20402

Wheat Flour Institute
14 East Jackson Blvd.
Chicago, IL 60604

WHO Publications Center USA
49 Sheridan Avenue
Albany, NY 12210

Wisconsin Association for Perinatal Care
McConnell Hall
1010 Mounds Street
Madison, WI 53715

TRANSPARENCY MASTERS

To make transparencies, insert acetate paper in place of typing paper into a photocopier machine. Acetate paper is easily obtained from companies selling paper and office supplies. It is often helpful for instruction purposes to write directly on overhead transparencies. Transparency pens can be purchased which are intended for this use. Notes made using transparency pens can then be rinsed off the transparency for future class use.

Chapter	Transparency Number	Description
Introduction	1	Factors that Promote Good Health
	2	Basic Functions of Nutrients and Oxygen
Chapter 1	3	Types of Vegetarian Diets
	4	Nutritious Menu Including Fast Foods
Chapter 2	5	Strategies to Promote Patient Discussion of Health Issues
	6	Active Listening Assessment Questions
Chapter 3	7	Anatomy of a Whole Grain
	8	Approximate Fiber Content of Foods
	9	Macronutrient Content of Major Food Groups Based on the Exchange System
Chapter 4	10	The Digestive System
Chapter 5	11	The Progression of Vitamin Deficiencies
	12	The pH of Body Fluids
Chapter 6	13	A Food Label
Chapter 7	14	Measuring Mid-upper Arm Circumference and Triceps Skinfold Thickness
	15	Sample Nutritional Assessment and Care Plan
Chapter 8	16	Recommended Total Fat for Various Kilocalorie Levels
	17	The Atherosclerosis Process
Chapter 9	18	Common Symptoms that Signal Hypoglycemia
	19	Hyperglycemia Versus Hypoglycemia
	20	Blood Glucose Curves: Reactive Hypoglycemia, Diabetes, and Normal Blood Sugars
	21	Insulin Regimens
Chapter 10	22	Dietary Guidelines and Modification for Renal Management
	23	Anatomy of a Kidney

Chapter	Transparency Number	Description
Chapter 11	24	Low Residue Diet as Modified with Food Groups from the Food Guide Pyramid
	25	Hiatal Hernia
	26	Preventing Constipation with a High Fiber Diet
	27	Preventing Diverticular Disease with a High Fiber Diet
Chapter 12	28	Pathways of Cancer Cachexia
	29	Surgical Procedures Requiring Postoperative Dietary Modifications
Chapter 13	30	Assessment of Protein Status
Chapter 14	31	Determination of Appropriate Nutritional Support
	32	Tube Feeding Routes
	33	TPN Insertion Route
Chapter 15	34	Common Correlations of Anorexia
Chapter 16	35	Fetal Development
	36	Components of Weight Gain During Pregnancy
	37	Recommended Prenatal Weight Gain Grid
	38	Milk Release During Breast-feeding
Chapter 17	39	Sample Growth Fall from Normal Curve
Chapter 18	40	Nutritional Goals for the Developmentally Disabled
	41	Proper Positioning for Mealtimes
	42	Assistive Devices for Eating Problems
Chapter 19	43	Good Snack Foods for Dental Health
Chapter 20	44	Dieting Tips
Chapter 21	45	DETERMINE Checklist
Chapter 22	46	Money-saving Food Shopping Skills
	47	Temperature Guide for Safe Storing of Food

TABLE 1   FACTORS THAT PROMOTE GOOD HEALTH

Good Diet
Eating right kind and amounts of food
Regular meals
Avoiding alcohol
Drinking adequate water

Good Mental Attitude
Positive outlook on life
Emotional stability
Social support group
Stress reduction

Regular Aerobic Exercise
Sufficient sleep and rest

Good Personal Hygiene and Habits
Not smoking
Good posture
Preventive care of teeth
Knowledge of and regular practice of self
    checks for disease warnings

Regular Medical Care
Recommended immunizations
Needed eye and ear examinations
Early attention to warning signs of disease

VITAMINS AND MINERALS =
THE GLUE THAT HOLDS BODY
CELLS (bricks) TOGETHER
(as represented by the
mortar and cement)

PROTEIN = BUILDING BLOCKS
(as represented by bricks)

WATER PROVIDES MOISTURE
AND PREVENTS DEHYDRATION
(as represented by the
kettle containing water)

OXYGEN AS FOUND IN AIR
IS NEEDED TO BURN FOOD
CALORIES FOR ENERGY
(as represented by air
circulating through the
chimney)

CARBOHYDRATES AND FAT
PROVIDE ENERGY AND HEAT
(as represented by the
burning wood/coal fire)

STORED ENERGY = BODY FAT
(represented by the coal bin
and wood pile)

COAL BIN

TYPES OF VEGETARIAN DIETS

1. *Lacto-ovo vegetarian.* Plant foods are supplemented with dairy products and eggs. This is probably the most common type of vegetarian diet. Lacto comes from the word lactose (milk sugar) and ovo comes from ovum or egg. Lacto-ovo vegetarians often also eat fish and chicken.

2. *Lacto-vegetarian.* Dairy products are included, but eggs are not.

3. *Total vegetarian (vegan).* Animal food sources (including both eggs and dairy products) are completely excluded. For this reason, this diet is likely to be low or inadequate in iodine, vitamin B_{12}, iron, calcium, zinc, riboflavin, and vitamin D.

NUTRITIOUS MENU INCLUDING FAST FOODS

Breakfast (At home)

Toasted English muffin with peanut butter

Banana slices dipped in wheat germ

Glass of low-fat or skim milk

Lunch (Cafeteria)

Chili con carne

Piece of cornbread

Glass of low-fat milk

Bunch of grapes (brought from home)

Supper (Fast food restaurant)

Small cheeseburger

Small orange juice

Large tossed salad with 1 tbsp regular dressing or free use of lemon juice or low-kilocalorie dressing

Snack (At home)

Herb-seasoned, low-fat popcorn

Apple cider

STRATEGIES TO PROMOTE PATIENT DISCUSSION OF HEALTH ISSUES

- **Use a warm, friendly, positive approach**

- **Sit in a comfortable proximity, neither too close nor too far away**

- **Use good eye-contact, with eyes intent but not staring**

- **Face the patient and lean forward**

- **Have arms unfolded and resting in a relaxed manner**

- **Carefully listen to what the patient is saying, using affirming comments to encourage the patient to clarify comments made**

- **Allow pauses in the conversation; take as long a pause as needed to consider how to best make replies—it shows you are interested in giving correct replies**

ACTIVE LISTENING ASSESSMENT QUESTIONS

How do you feel about _____?

Can you tell me what you know about _____?

Is _____ a problem for your family?

Can you tell me more about _____?

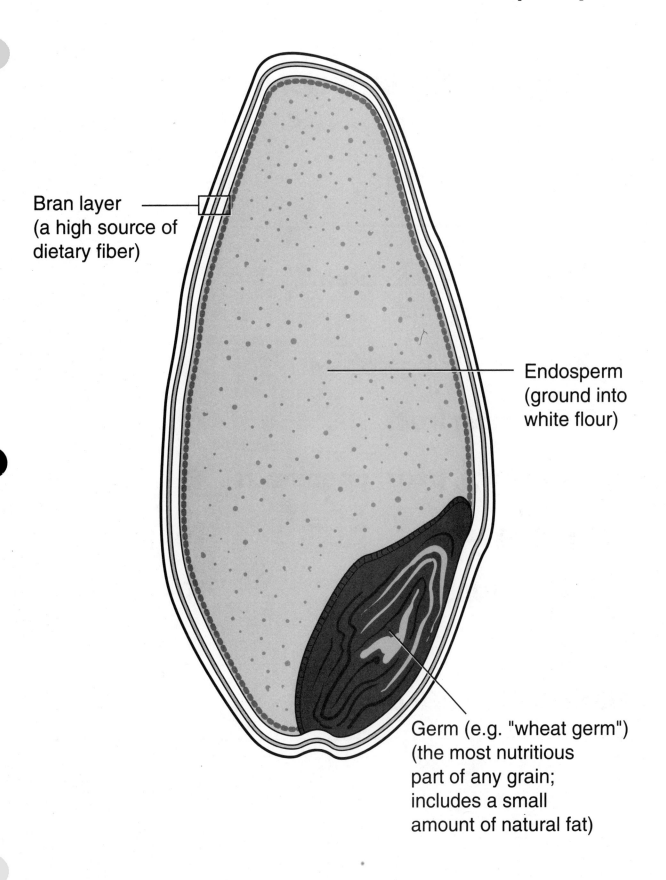

Bran layer
(a high source of
dietary fiber)

Endosperm
(ground into
white flour)

Germ (e.g. "wheat germ")
(the most nutritious
part of any grain;
includes a small
amount of natural fat)

APPROXIMATE FIBER CONTENT OF FOODS

	GRAMS OF FIBER
1 Slice whole-grain bread/ grain products	**2**
1/2 Cup most vegetables	**2**
1/2 Cup most fruits	**2**
1/2 Cup corn, peas, or spinach	**5**
1/2 Cup legumes	**10**
1/2 Cup bran cereals	**10–15**
FIBER GOALS PER DAY:	**20–30**

MACRONUTRIENT CONTENT OF MAJOR FOOD GROUPS BASED ON THE EXCHANGE SYSTEM

Grain group	15 g carbohydrate
	3 g protein
Vegetable group	5 g carbohydrate
	2 g protein
Fruit group	15 g carbohydrate
Milk group	12 g carbohydrate
	8 g protein
	10 g fat (whole milk)
	5 g fat (2% milk)
	2 g fat (1% milk)
	0 g fat (skim milk)
Meat group	7 g protein
	5 g fat
	8–10 g fat (high-fat choices)
	1–2 g fat (lean meat choices)

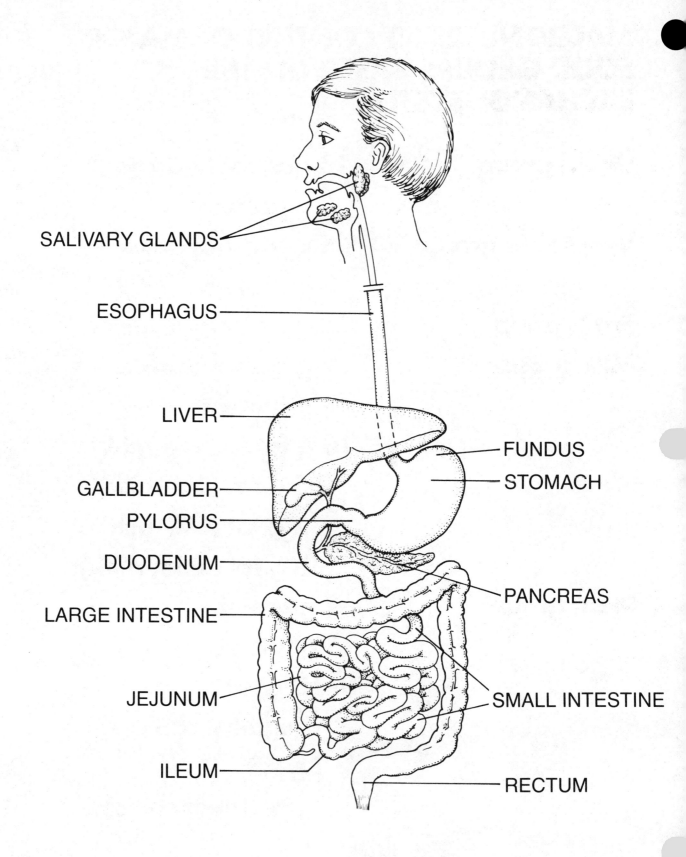

SALIVARY GLANDS

ESOPHAGUS

LIVER

FUNDUS

STOMACH

GALLBLADDER

PYLORUS

DUODENUM

PANCREAS

LARGE INTESTINE

JEJUNUM

SMALL INTESTINE

ILEUM

RECTUM

SEVERE DEFICIENCY
Appearance of clinical signs of deficiency disease

MILD DEFICIENCY
Abnormal biochemical, blood, and urine tests

DIETARY DEFICIENCY
Inadequate intake of a vitamin from food sources

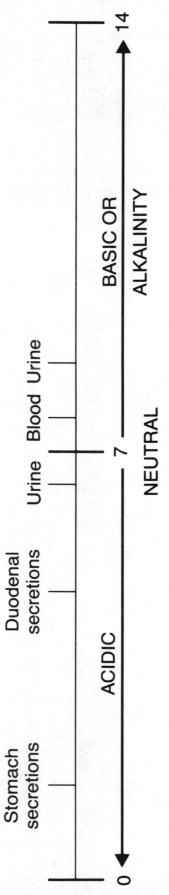

The New Food Label at a Glance

Nutrition Facts

Serving Size 1 cup (228g)
Servings Per Container 2

Amount Per Serving

Calories 260   Calories from Fat 120

% Daily Value*

Total Fat 13g	**20**%
Saturated Fat 5g	**25**%
Cholesterol 30mg	**10**%
Sodium 660mg	**28**%
Total Carbohydrate 31g	**10**%
Dietary Fiber 0g	**0**%
Sugars 5g	
Protein 5g	

Vitamin A 4%	•	Vitamin C 2%	
Calcium 15%	•	Iron 4%	

---

* Percent Daily Values are based on a 2,000 calorie diet. Your daily values may be higher or lower depending on your calorie needs:

	Calories:	2,000	2,500
Total Fat	Less than	65g	80g
Sat Fat	Less than	20g	25g
Cholesterol	Less than	300mg	300mg
Sodium	Less than	2,400mg	2,400mg
Total Carbohydrate		300g	375g
Dietary Fiber		25g	30g

Calories per gram:
Fat 9 • Carbohydrate 4 • Protein 4

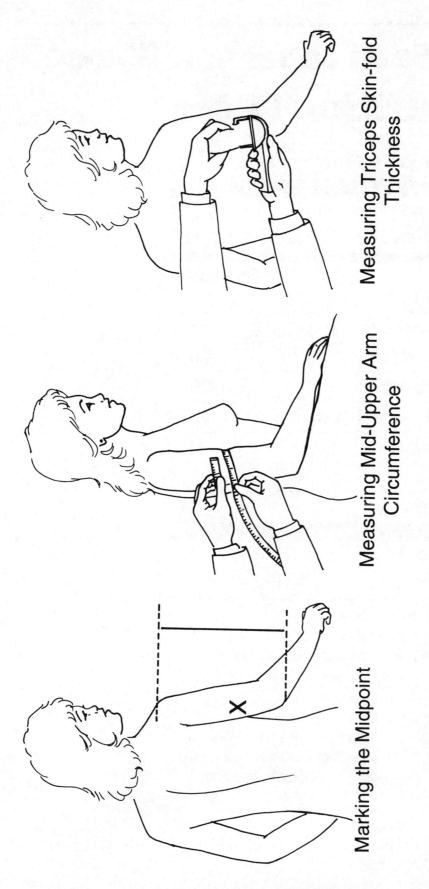

Measuring Triceps Skin-fold Thickness

Measuring Mid-Upper Arm Circumference

Marking the Midpoint

Name _____ Date of Birth _____ Male/Female

Diet Prescription_____ Diagnosis _____

Activity Level _____ Appetite _____

Medications

Meal Pattern

B   L   S

Food Preferences: Food Intolerances/Dislikes:

_____

Clinical Data : Skin Condition_____ Edema _____

Impairments: Eyesight _____Hearing _____ Speech _____Taste _____

       Chewing and Swallowing Ability_____

Present Weight___Usual Weight_____ Desired Weight Range_____

Elbow Breadth___Midarm Circumference___Triceps Skin Fold____

Height _____

Meal Observation: Percentage of food consumed __ Fluid intake__mL

       Type of assistance needed _____

       Affective response to food _____

Biochemical Data:

Serum laboratory values:_____

_____

Urinalysis: _____

Skin Tests: _____

Evaluation and Recommendation: _____

Problem/Need	Intervention	By Whom	Goal	Response/Date

By: _____   Title: _____

Date: _____

TABLE 8-4 RECOMMENDED TOTAL FAT FOR VARIOUS KILOCALORIE LEVELS

Kilocalorie Level	Total Recommended Fat (30%)
1200 kilocalories	40 g fat
1500 kilocalories	50 g fat
1800 kilocalories	60 g fat
2100 kilocalories	70 g fat
2400 kilocalories	80 g fat
2700 kilocalories	90 g fat
3000 kilocalories	100 g fat

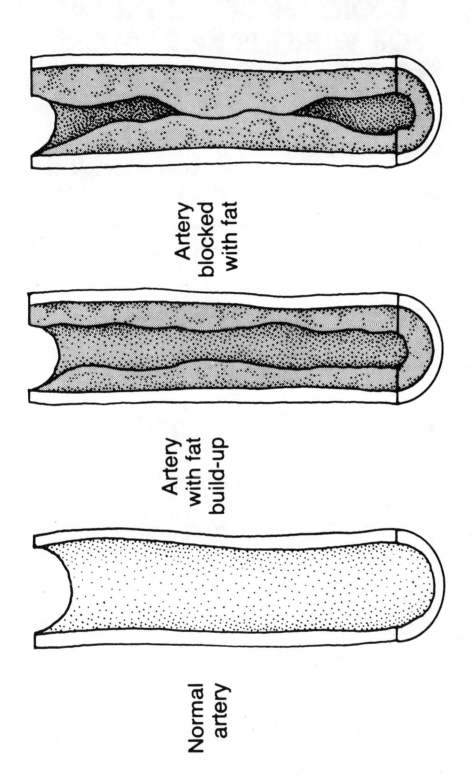

Artery blocked with fat

Artery with fat build-up

Normal artery

TABLE 9-4 COMMON SYMPTOMS THAT SIGNAL HYPOGLYCEMIA

- Clammy skin
- Mental confusion
- Physical tremor
- Weakness
- Headache
- Rapid heart beat
- Double or blurred vision

HYPOGLYCEMIA
(Excess insulin causes too much transport of glucose from the blood.)

TISSUE CELLS

BLOOD GLUCOSE

CARBOHYDRATE DIGESTION

HYPERGLYCEMIA
(Inadequate availability of insulin for glucose transport causes glucose to build up in the blood stream.)

TISSUE CELLS

BLOOD GLUCOSE

CARBOHYDRATE DIGESTION

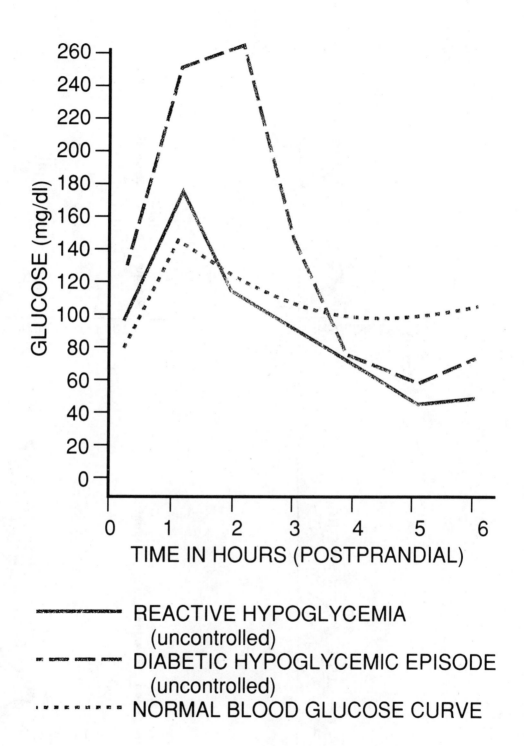

TIME IN HOURS (POSTPRANDIAL)

—————— REACTIVE HYPOGLYCEMIA
(uncontrolled)

– – – – DIABETIC HYPOGLYCEMIC EPISODE
(uncontrolled)

· · · · · · · · NORMAL BLOOD GLUCOSE CURVE

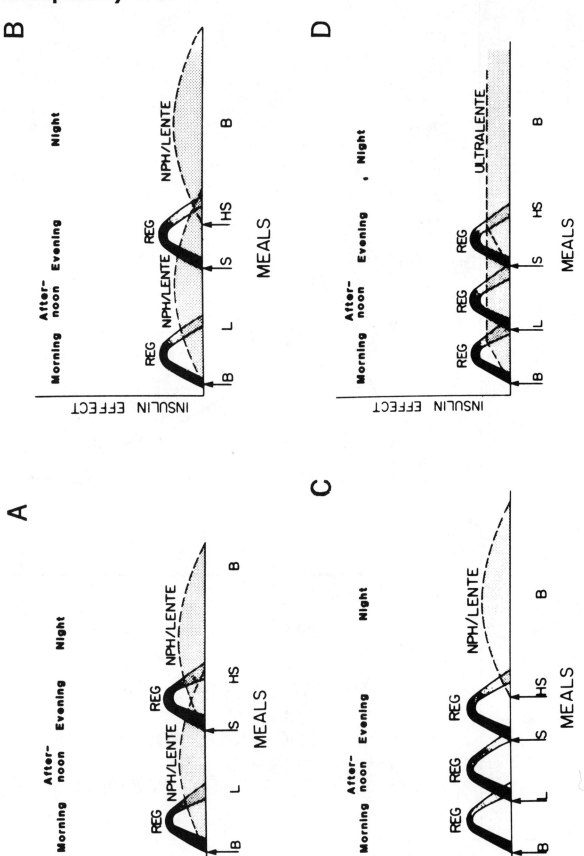

TABLE 11-6   LOW RESIDUE DIET AS MODIFIED WITH FOOD GROUPS FROM THE FOOD GUIDE PYRAMID

Grains	**Emphasize refined grain products such as white bread, white rice, pasta, and cereals that are not whole grain**
Vegetables/fruits	**Emphasize those without skins or seeds such as canned fruits and fruit juice**
Milk	**Two cups or more as tolerated**
Meat	**Emphasize tender meats; avoid fried meats or those with gristle**
	Avoid legumes and nuts

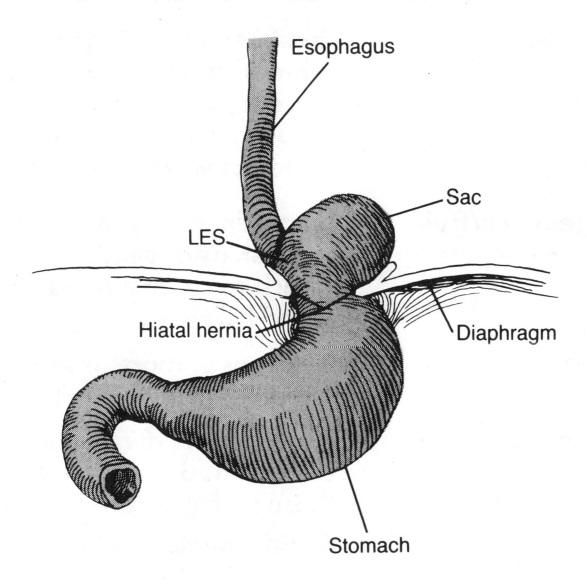

Esophagus

Sac

LES

Hiatal hernia

Diaphragm

Stomach

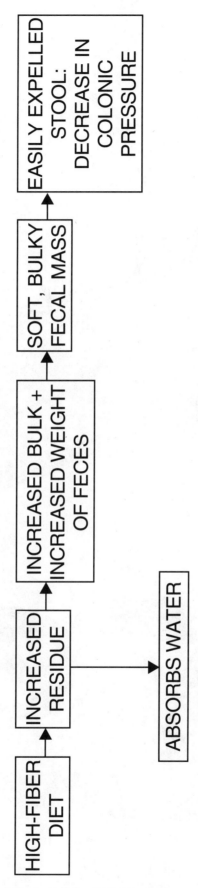

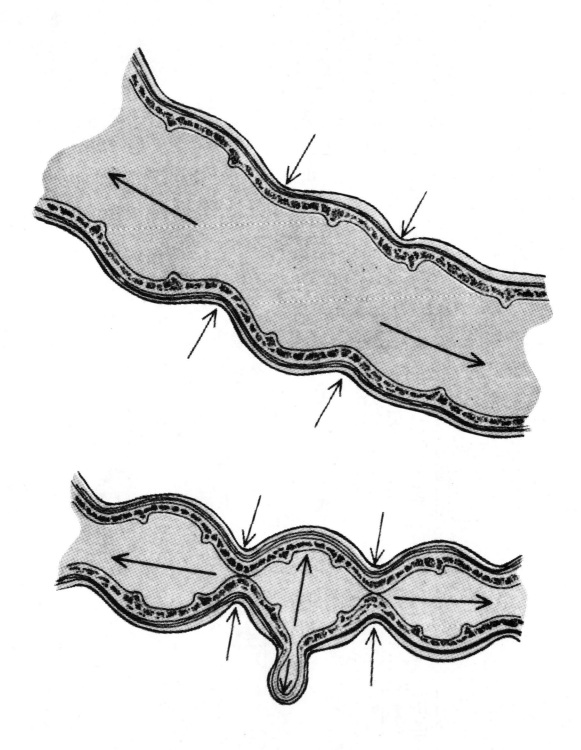

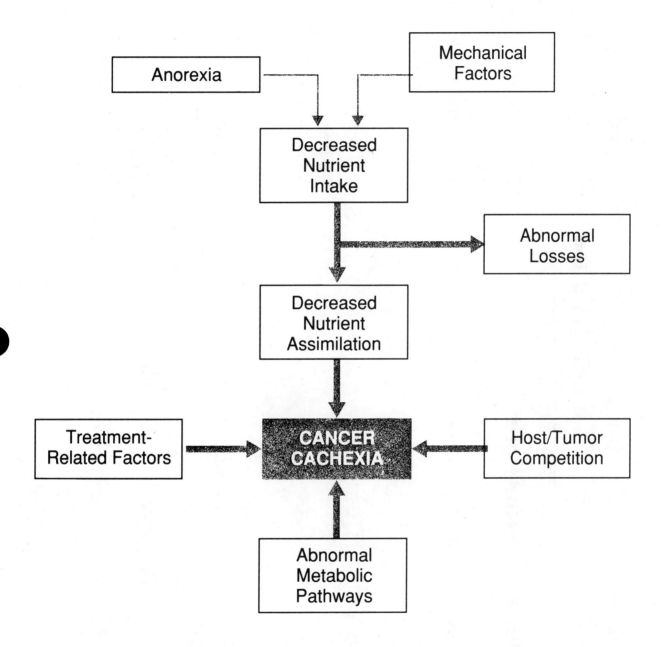

TABLE 12-4

SURGICAL PROCEDURES REQUIRING POSTOPERATIVE DIETARY MODIFICATIONS

Procedure	Nutritional Problems	Dietary Modifications
Radical neck resection	Inability to chew or swallow	Nasogastric tube feeding
Gastrectomy	"Dumping syndrome"	Small frequent meals, liquids between meals, restrict concentrated carbohydrate
Small bowel resection	Diarrhea, malabsorption	Elemental diet
Ileostomy; colostomy	Fluid and electrolyte imbalances	Replacement of fluids and electrolytes

Protein status can be determined through:

- **anthropometric measurements such as weight for height, percent weight loss from usual or last recorded weight, tricep skinfold measures, and mid-arm circumference**

- **lab values such as serum albumin level**

- **a diet history, which can determine if the diet contains adequate amounts of protein**

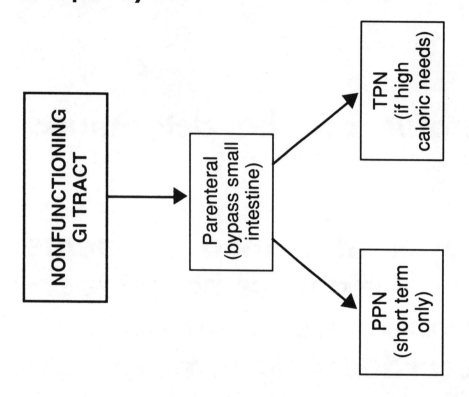

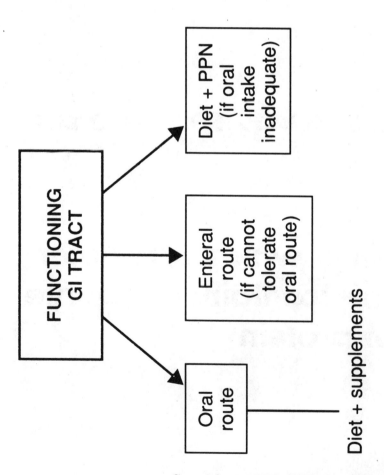

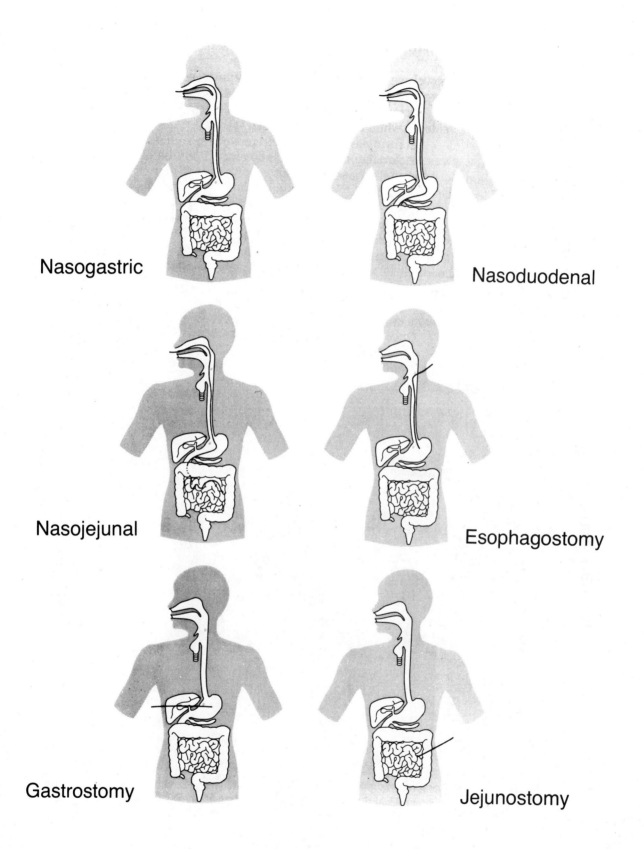

Nasogastric

Nasoduodenal

Nasojejunal

Esophagostomy

Gastrostomy

Jejunostomy

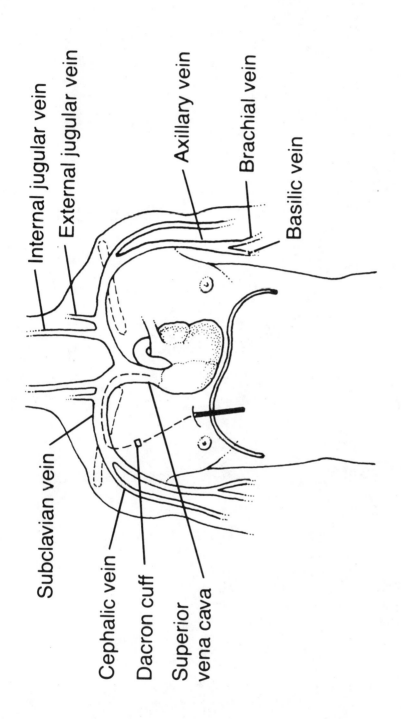

Internal jugular vein
External jugular vein
Axillary vein
Brachial vein
Basilic vein
Subclavian vein
Cephalic vein
Dacron cuff
Superior vena cava

COMMON CORRELATIONS OF ANOREXIA

- The person with anorexia nervosa has an intense fear of becoming obese that does not lessen as weight loss progresses.

- There is a disturbance of body image, such as claiming to feel fat even when emaciated.

- There is a weight loss of at least 25 per cent of original body weight.

- There is refusal to maintain body weight over a minimal healthy weight for age and height.

- There is no known physical illness that would account for the weight loss.

- Amenorrhea results in girls due to altered hormonal states.

- Bizarre eating habits are observed such as cutting food into tiny pieces or limiting intake to only a few foods.

- An underlying low self-esteem is common among persons with anorexia.

- Compulsive exercise habits may also be found in anorexia.

TABLE 16-1   FETAL DEVELOPMENT

First Trimester (Embryo; Critical Stage)	Second Trimester (Fetus)	Third Trimester to Birth
Organs develop (4–12 weeks)	Growth and development continue (13-40 weeks)	Growth and development continue
Central nervous system develops (4-12 weeks)	Teeth calcify (20 weeks)	Storage of iron and other nutrients (36–40 weeks; premature babies often deficient in iron)
Skeletal structure hardens from cartilage to bone (4 weeks)	Fetus can survive outside womb (24 weeks)	Development of necessary fat tissue (36-40 weeks)

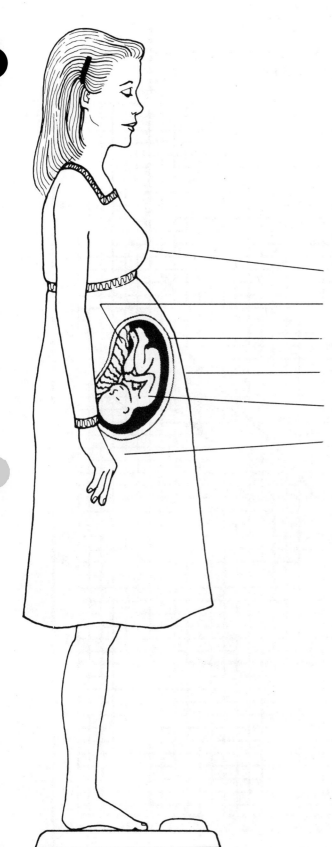

Your baby accounts for only part
of the weight you must gain

1 lb., breasts

1½ lb., placenta (afterbirth)

2 lb., uterus

8½ lb., increased blood and fluids

7½ lb., baby

3½ lb., mother's stores

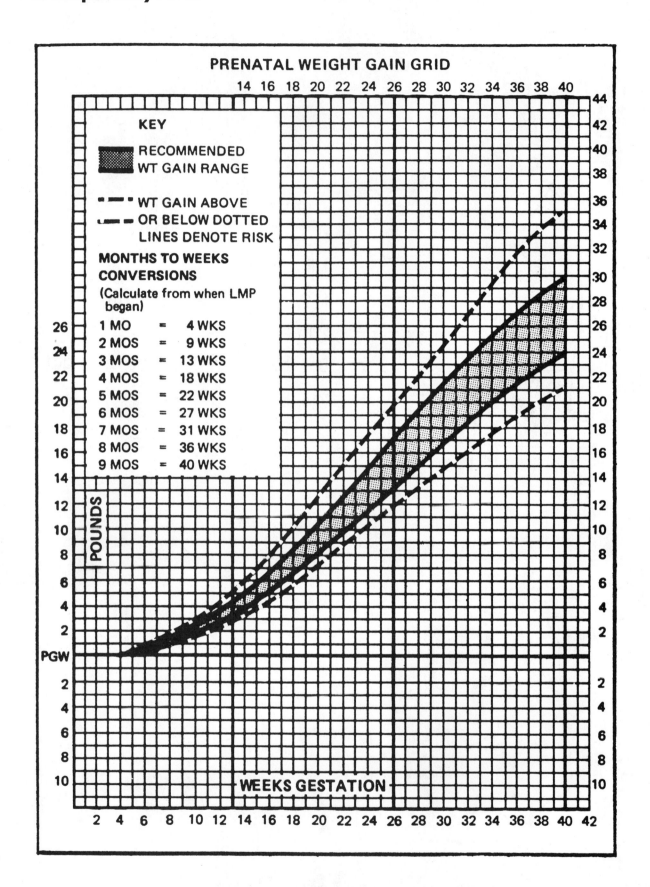

PRENATAL WEIGHT GAIN GRID

KEY

RECOMMENDED WT GAIN RANGE

WT GAIN ABOVE OR BELOW DOTTED LINES DENOTE RISK

MONTHS TO WEEKS CONVERSIONS
(Calculate from when LMP began)

1 MO	=	4 WKS
2 MOS	=	9 WKS
3 MOS	=	13 WKS
4 MOS	=	18 WKS
5 MOS	=	22 WKS
6 MOS	=	27 WKS
7 MOS	=	31 WKS
8 MOS	=	36 WKS
9 MOS	=	40 WKS

POUNDS

PGW

WEEKS GESTATION

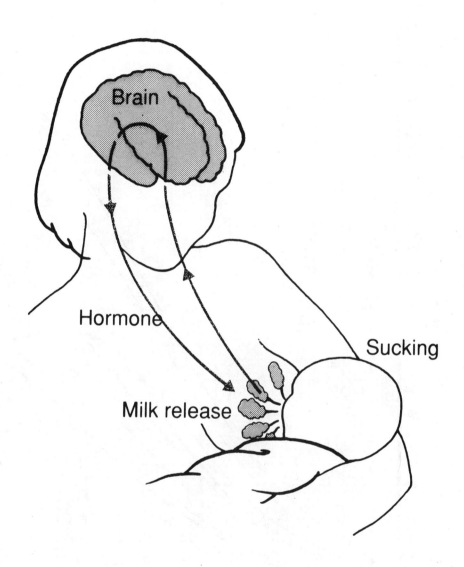

Brain

Hormone

Milk release

Sucking

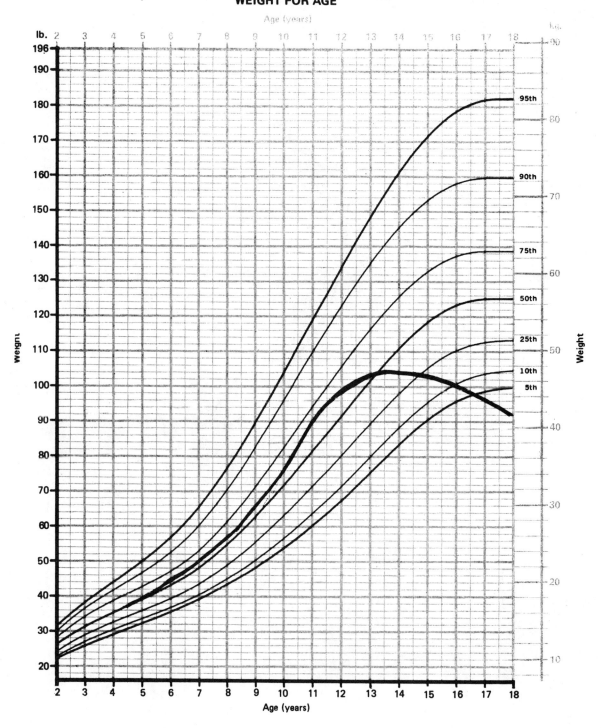

GIRLS FROM 2 TO 18 YEARS
WEIGHT FOR AGE

DEVELOPMENTAL DISABILITIES

Mental Retardation
Autism
Cerebral Palsy
Neurological Impairment
Epilepsy
Others

NUTRITIONAL PROBLEMS

Growth Retardation
Dehydration
Food Allergy or Intolerance
Constipation
Drug-Nutrient Interactions
Eating Problems
Obesity

GOALS

Weight Control
Hydration
Drooling Control
Eating Independence
Improved Sucking Reflex
Adequate Nutrient and
Kilocalorie Intake
Improved Chewing and
Swallowing Pattern

INTERVENTIONS

Diet Modification
(nutrients, calories, consistency)
Behavioral Management
Increased Exercise
Nutrient Supplementation
Individual Training and Counseling
Care Provider Counseling
Use of Assistive Devices

WRONG

RIGHT

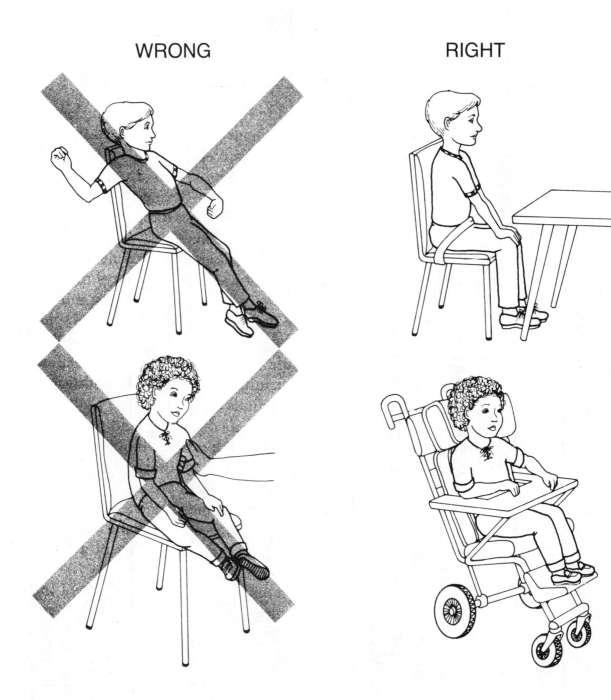

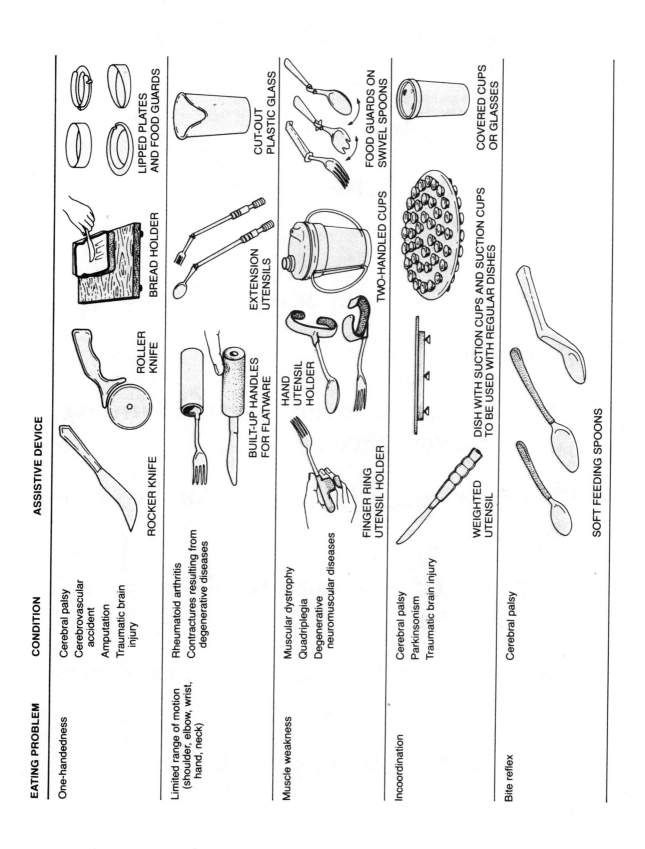

EATING PROBLEM	CONDITION	ASSISTIVE DEVICE
One-handedness	Cerebral palsy Cerebrovascular accident Amputation Traumatic brain injury	ROCKER KNIFE, ROLLER KNIFE, BREAD HOLDER LIPPED PLATES AND FOOD GUARDS CUT-OUT PLASTIC GLASS
Limited range of motion (shoulder, elbow, wrist, hand, neck)	Rheumatoid arthritis Contractures resulting from degenerative diseases	BUILT-UP HANDLES FOR FLATWARE EXTENSION UTENSILS
Muscle weakness	Muscular dystrophy Quadriplegia Degenerative neuromuscular diseases	HAND UTENSIL HOLDER FINGER RING UTENSIL HOLDER TWO-HANDLED CUPS FOOD GUARDS ON SWIVEL SPOONS
Incoordination	Cerebral palsy Parkinsonism Traumatic brain injury	WEIGHTED UTENSIL DISH WITH SUCTION CUPS AND SUCTION CUPS TO BE USED WITH REGULAR DISHES COVERED CUPS OR GLASSES
Bite reflex	Cerebral palsy	SOFT FEEDING SPOONS

GOOD SNACK FOODS FOR DENTAL HEALTH

- **Carrot and celery sticks**

- **Zucchini "matchsticks"**

- **Radishes**

- **Green and red pepper rings**

- **Cucumber slices**

- **Peanuts and other nuts (for children over 3 years to avoid choking)**

- **Cheese, regular in moderation or low-fat varieties**

- **Hard-cooked egg, with or without the yolk (for cholesterol control)**

- **Grain products (crackers, toast, bagels) with peanut butter or cheese**

- **Apple wedges with peanut butter**

- **Milk or yogurt**

TABLE 20-2   DIETING TIPS

1. Eat regularly, choosing foods low in fat and sugar.
2. Chew thoroughly and slowly.
3. Stop eating when the stomach is comfortably full.
4. Make diet changes that can be maintained for life; temporary quick fixes are counter-productive for healthy weight management.
5. Wait 15 minutes before having second helpings.
6. Include exercise for healthy weight management.
7. To deal with the "clean your plate" practice, remember that excess food goes either to waste or to the waist.
8. When faced with an indulgence, ask yourself "How will I feel tomorrow if I don't eat this food today?" Give yourself permission to eat if feelings of deprivation may arise.
9. When ready to give up on dieting efforts, remember Ann Landers' quote, "The difference between a successful person and an unsuccessful person is that the successful person never stops trying."
10. For individualized meal-planning tips, consult a registered dietitian, the expert in nutrition.

Disease

Eating Poorly

Tooth Loss/ Mouth Pain

Economic Hardship

Reduced Social Contact

Mutiple Medicines

Involuntary Weight Loss/Gain

Needs Assistance in Self Care

Elder Years Above Age 80

TABLE 22-6   MONEY-SAVING FOOD SHOPPING SKILLS

- Use less tender cuts of meat, which are less expensive. To tenderize, cook slowly with moisture (such as in stews) or grind, cube, or pound the meat. Marinating in an acid such as lemon or tomato juice also helps to tenderize meat.

- Extend meat, poultry, and fish by making casseroles using legumes (dried beans), pasta, rice, or potatoes.

- Include meatless meals once or twice a week using legumes, eggs, cheese, or peanut butter in its place for protein.

- Buy in bulk whenever possible and freeze as needed.

- Study unit pricing to determine the best buy per pound or ounce.

- Take advantage of specials and use coupons.

- Try lower-priced, "generic" store brands, which are often of similar quality to more expensive brands.

- Plan meals to include leftovers.

- Shop for low-cost foods within each food group.

- Use food labels to compare nutritional value for cost to get your money's worth.

Transparency # 47

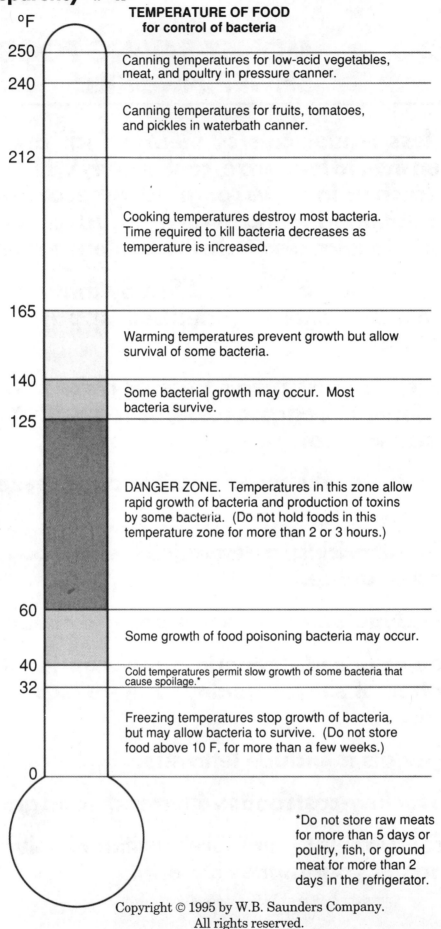

°F

TEMPERATURE OF FOOD
for control of bacteria

250 — Canning temperatures for low-acid vegetables, meat, and poultry in pressure canner.

240 —

Canning temperatures for fruits, tomatoes, and pickles in waterbath canner.

212 —

Cooking temperatures destroy most bacteria. Time required to kill bacteria decreases as temperature is increased.

165 —

Warming temperatures prevent growth but allow survival of some bacteria.

140 — Some bacterial growth may occur. Most bacteria survive.

125 —

DANGER ZONE. Temperatures in this zone allow rapid growth of bacteria and production of toxins by some bacteria. (Do not hold foods in this temperature zone for more than 2 or 3 hours.)

60 —

Some growth of food poisoning bacteria may occur.

40 — Cold temperatures permit slow growth of some bacteria that cause spoilage.*

32 —

Freezing temperatures stop growth of bacteria, but may allow bacteria to survive. (Do not store food above 10 F. for more than a few weeks.)

0 —

*Do not store raw meats for more than 5 days or poultry, fish, or ground meat for more than 2 days in the refrigerator.